WM18   BELL LIBRARY

D1633542

NX00001926

Get Through

MRCPsych

Prepa   C

Second Edition

Sree Prathap Mohana Murthy MB BS, MRCPsych
Hertfordshire Partnership NHS Trust

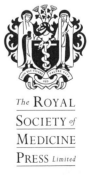

The ROYAL
SOCIETY *of*
MEDICINE
PRESS *Limited*

© 2008 Royal Society of Medicine Ltd

Published by the Royal Society of Medicine Press Ltd
1 Wimpole Street, London W1G 0AE, UK
Tel: +44 (0)20 7290 2921
Fax: +44 (0)20 7290 2929
E-mail: publishing@rsmpress.co.uk

Apart from any fair dealing for the purposes of research or private study,
criticism or review, as permitted under the UK Copyright, Designs and Patents
Act, 1988, no part of this publication may be reproduced, stored or transmitted,
in any form or by any means without the prior permission in writing of the
publishers or, in the case of reprographic reproduction, in accordance with the
terms of licences issued by the Copyright Licensing Reproduction Rights
Organization outside the UK. Enquiries concerning reproduction outside the terms
stated here should be sent to the publishers at the UK address printed on this
page.

The right of Sree Prathap Mohana Murthy to be identified as author of this work
has been asserted by him in accordance with the Copyright, Designs and Patents
Act, 1988.

British Library Cataloguing in Publication Data
A catalogue record for this book is available from the British Library

ISBN: 978-1-85315-876-6

Distribution in Europe and Rest of the World:
Marston Book Services Ltd
PO Box 269
Abingdon
Oxon OX14 4YN, UK
Tel: +44 (0)1235 465500
Fax: +44 (0)1235 465555
Email: direct.order@marston.co.uk

Distribution in USA and Canada:
Royal Society of Medicine Press Ltd
C/o BookMasters Inc
30 Amberwood Parkway
Ashland, OH 44805, USA
Tel: +1 800 247 6553/ +1 800 266 5564
Fax: +1 410 281 6883
Email: order@bookmasters.com

Distribution in Australia and New Zealand:
Elsevier Australia
30–52 Smidmore Street
Marrickville NSW 2204, Australia
Tel: +61 2 9517 8999
Fax: +61 2 9517 2249
nail: service@elsevier.com.au

I   neset by Phoenix Photosetting, Chatham, Kent
         the UK by Bell & Bain Ltd, Glasgow

Contents

BELL LIBRARY WMI
NEW CROSS HOSPITAL
WOLVERHAMPTON
Tel: 01902 695322

Introduction   v
About the Author   vii
Essential tips for CASC (Clinical assessment of skills and competencies) ix

Risk assessment
Suicide   3
Puerperal Disorder   9
Violence   13

History Taking and Symptom Elicitation
Alcohol History   19
Illicit Drug History   24
Eating Disorder History   28
Symptoms of Depression   32
Hallucinations   36
First-rank Symptoms   40
Delusions and other Experiences   44
Manic Symptoms   48
Anxiety Symptoms   52
Post-Traumatic Stress Disorder (PTSD) History   55
Obsessive–Compulsive Disorder Symptoms   59
Assessing Insight   62
Mental State Examination   63
Premorbid Personality   66
Dementia – Obtaining Collateral History   69

Counselling/Explanation about a Particular Disease or Condition
Schizophrenia   79
Bipolar Affective Disorder   87
Depression   95
Postnatal Depression   100
Alcohol – Problems, Risks and Motivation   104
Alzheimer's Disease   108

Counselling/Explanation about a Particular Drug or Treatment
Electroconvulsive Therapy to the Patient   115
Treatment with Atypical Antipsychotics   120
Clozapine Treatment   125
Antidepressant Treatment (Selective Serotonin Re-uptake Inhibitors)   132
Lithium Carbonate   138
Valproate Semisodium   143
Antidementia Drugs – Explain to a Carer
Depot Medication   152

iii

Cognitive Behavioural Therapy 158
Obsessive–Compulsive Disorder and Treatment Options 161
Treatment Options for Agoraphobia 165
Panic Disorder and Hyperventilation Syndrome 167

Examinations
Mini-mental State Examination 173
Perform Detailed Cognitive Examination 176
Frontal Lobe Function Testing 180
Parietal Lobe Function Testing 182
Extrapyramidal Side Effects – Physical Examination 184
Cranial Nerves 186
Thyroid Gland 189
Sensory and Motor Examination of Upper Limbs 192
Sensory and Motor Examination of Lower Limbs 195
Cardiovascular System 198
Gastrointestinal System 200
Respiratory System 203
Alcohol Misuse – Physical Examination 206
Opiate Withdrawal – Physical Examination 209
Eating Disorder – Physical Examination 211
ECT – Electrode Placement 213
ECG Recording 215
Interpretation of ECG 217
Cardiopulmonary Resuscitation (CPR) 220
Fundoscopy 222

Interpretation of Blood Results and Management
Neuroleptic Malignant Syndrome 227
Serotonin Syndrome 230
Eating Disorder 232

Miscellaneous Topics
Rapid Tranquillization 241
Telephone Advice About a Confused Patient 245
Assess Capacity 247
Discharge Arrangements 250

References 253

Introduction

The MRCPsych Clinical Assessment of Skills and Competencies (CASC) exam is scheduled for introduction in Spring 2008 with the initial phased introduction, followed by full implementation in Autumn 2008.

The exam will comprise two parts, both to be completed in one day. There will be two types of circuits in the MRCPsych examination: one will include ten single or stand-alone stations; the other format will include five pairs of 'linked stations', where two stations are linked together to form a pair. This allows assessment of more 'advanced' clinical skills.

In simple stations, you have one minute to carefully read the instructions for each station, which are posted outside the station. Most instructions are brief. A bell will ring to indicate when you may enter the station. Each station lasts eight minutes and a one-minute warning will be given. Following the final bell, you must then stop the task and go and wait outside the next station.

The complex or linked stations will comprise linked pairs of stations with a clinical task in the first station which will be linked to a related task in the second station. Candidate instructions in the first station of each pair will state, in broad terms, what task should be carried out in the second station. Each station will consist of 2 minutes' preparation time followed by twelve minutes attempting the defined task. A one-minute warning will be given.

There will be an examiner in each station and you should only direct comments to the examiner if the examiner or the instructions specifically ask you to do so.

In the MRCPsych Examination, these stations consist of clinical scenarios set at a standard expected of an ST2–3 trainee. The scenarios in the exams aim to test candidates' competency in clinical skills appropriate to their stage of training.

The list of skills to be tested includes:

1. History taking
2. Counselling/offering explanation about a particular disease or drug
3. Clinical examination
4. Procedural skills
5. Risk assessment
6. Discussing treatment options for a particular condition
7. Telephone conversation
8. Discussing the management plan with the consultant.

Although you need to have a certain amount of knowledge to succeed in the CASC, it is important to realize that the exam is testing both clinical and communication skills. You need to be able to use your knowledge in a clinical setting, assessing patients by asking the right questions and reassuring patients appropriately, accurately and sensitively. Here, your attitude, confidence, and communication skills will be tested as well as your knowledge.

Reading textbooks alone will not help you pass the exam. You must polish your interview skills by talking to real patients and, ideally, your performance should be observed by a senior colleague who will offer constructive criticism.

This book contains stations/questions that have been encountered by candidates in the previous MRCPsych Part 1 OSCE examinations and also many other scenarios that might be important and are more likely to appear in future examinations.

I hope that this book will give you an overview of what the CASC exam is all about. The answers I have given should be used as a guide to form your own responses. Reference to standard textbooks is also recommended.

For those who might be interested in further learning and formulating management plans for common psychiatric conditions, please refer to my other book *Get Through Workplace Based Assessments in Psychiatry*. This is a fully revised edition of *Get Through MRCPsych Part 2: Clinical Exam: Long Case Presentations*.

Good luck!
Sree Prathap Mohana Murthy

About the Author

I am currently working at Hertfordshire Partnership NHS Trust, training to become an Old Age Psychiatrist. I did my undergraduate medical education in India and did my postgraduate training in Psychiatry at North Essex Mental Health Partnership NHS Trust, UK.

I received the prestigious Pfizer Award for the best performance in the final year examination during my undergraduate medical training. I also received the Dr. Venkoba Rao Gold Medal in Psychiatry for 1998 and also won first prize in the South Indian Level Psychiatric Quiz Competition in 1998.

I am very interested in teaching and run my own revision course for psychiatric trainees, The SPMM Course, based in London (www.spmmcourse.com). I organize revision courses for psychiatric trainees for both written papers and CASC examinations.

I have previously written two books entitled *Get Through MRCPsych Part 1: Preparation for the OSCEs*, and *Get Through MRCPsych Part 2: Clinical Exam: Long Case Presentations* both published by the RSM Press Ltd.

In line with the new exam format, I have fully revised *Get Through MRCPsych Part 2: Clinical Exam: Long Case Presentations* and this will be available shortly, entitled *Get Through Workplace Based Assessments in Psychiatry*, which I hope can be used as a handbook for all trainees in psychiatry who are involved in WPBAs.

Sree Prathap Mohana Murthy

This book is dedicated to
My beloved mother Mrs Kosalai Mohana Murthy
and
My beloved father Mr Mohana Murthy

Essential tips for CASC (Clinical assessment of skills and competencies)

Things that you should or should not do:

- **Weeks before the exam:** Reading textbooks alone will not help you pass the CASC. It is useful and makes sense to practice the clinical scenarios in small groups of 3–4. Do not rely solely on reading.

- **The day before the exam**: Take adequate rest and ensure that you get enough sleep the night before the exam.

- **On the day of the exam**, eat a good breakfast or lunch, adequate hydration is important.

- **Outside each station read the question properly**: Read instructions carefully. Stick to them.

- **On entering the booth:** When you enter the booth, give the examiner your candidate number. On entering the station, acknowledge the presence of the examiner by eye contact but then turn your attention to the patient and greet them politely.

- Set up the chairs as part of your first few seconds.

- Sit down before introducing yourself. However, if the patient is already standing, **introduce yourself** by shaking hands, ask the patient to take a seat and then sit down yourself. Your handshake should be quick and firm.

- As a general rule most people like to be addressed by their **surname**. If they prefer first name, they will tell you.

- Ensure your **body language** is both appropriate and under your control.

- Establish good **eye contact** and always appear confident, calm and in control of the situation. In short, be professional.

- At the **beginning** of the interview you must tell the patient what you are going to do in broad terms, and some of the topics that you intend to cover.

- Start with **Open** questions and then proceed to **Closed** questions.

- Always try to address patient's **concerns** first.

- Listen to what the patient says and try to **pick up clues** from what the patient tells you.

- Do not take too rigid an approach; you must be prepared to '**go with the flow**' and adapt to the situation.

- **If asked to give explanations:** Always elicit what the patient understands first.

- Respect patients' dignity, privacy and protect confidential information.

- Avoid using **complicated medical terms** unless absolutely necessary. Give information in a way the patient will understand.

- Avoid giving **false information** and avoid false reassurance. Be honest and trustworthy.

- **Before ending the interview:** Give the patient adequate opportunity to ask questions. Do not leave it until the last minute to interview them. As soon as you hear the warning bell, use that time to summarize and conclude the interview.

- If you finish early, spend a little time **reflecting** on what you have covered.

- At the end, it is worth mentioning useful sources of information such as leaflets, videotapes, websites, self-help groups, support groups and voluntary organizations.

- In **Physical examination** stations, in general, perfection is not expected. Before beginning the examination, explain to the patient clearly what you are going to do and give them clear instructions. Ask permission before you proceed. Ensure privacy and, for female patients, always request a chaperone. Be considerate and gentle when examining patients.

- Do not forget to thank the patient and examiner before leaving.

- Outside the station, do not become distracted by thinking about the station you have just completed – **focus on the next station.**

- During rest stations, stay calm. Use rest stations to think ahead not backwards.

- Most importantly, everyone has his or her own interview style, do not change what works well for you.

Risk Assessment

SUICIDE

Task: Assess the current risk of suicide in Miss Vicky Smith, a young woman admitted to the medical ward following an overdose.

Suicide risk assessment has usually been asked as a paired/complex station, where in the first station you will be asked to do a risk assessment, and in the next station you have to discuss with the consultant, over the phone, about the assessment done and your further management plan.

Suicide risk assessment: Areas to concentrate on:

- Obtain more information about the overdose.
- Evaluate the degree of suicidal intent and seriousness of the attempt.
- Investigate symptoms of depression/psychosis or other forms of mental illness.
- Assess current mental state including suicidal thoughts.
- Take past history and background information.
- Assess coping methods and ability to seek help.

Suggested approach

- Greet the patient and introduce yourself.
- Explain the purpose of the visit.
- Obtain permission before you proceed.
- Use open questions to give the patient an adequate opportunity to ventilate their feelings.
- The patient may be distressed and therefore try to acknowledge her distress.
- Allow her to speak freely, noting her concerns. This may help relieve tension and allow you to assess her mental state.

Step 1: Obtain the following information about the overdose

1. How many tablets were taken?
2. What type of tablets were taken?
3. When was the overdose taken?
4. How was the medication obtained?
5. Where was the patient when she took the overdose?

6. How and by whom was she discovered?

7. What did she do after the overdose?

8. How did she end up coming to hospital?

9. Did she take anything else with the tablets, for example, alcohol?

10. Why did she take the overdose? (or)

- What was the event leading up to the suicidal act? (or)

- What made her think of harming herself? (or)

- What sorts of things had been worrying her?

If the patient is not forthcoming with all the details, use more closed questions and also examples like:

- Conflict in a close relationship

- A major loss or separation

- Family disharmony

- Difficulties at work

- Financial worries/housing

- Health problems

- Redundancy or legal problems

- Was there any direct gain? (e.g. was the patient in custody at the time of the act?)

Step 2: Assessment of the degree of suicidal intent and seriousness of the attempt

A detailed assessment should include evaluation of the characteristics of the attempt:

Remember 4 Ps:
1. Planning/impulsivity

2. Performance in isolation or in front of others

3. Preparations made prior to the act

4. Precautions to avoid discovery by others.

Questions

A. Degree of suicidal intent

- Did the person plan the attempt carefully or was it impulsive?

- Did she take any steps towards doing this? (e.g. getting pills)
- Was anyone else actually present at the time?
- Did she convey her suicidal intent to others?
- Where did the act take place?
- Would she have anticipated being found?
- Did she take measures to avoid discovery?
- Did she make any preparations like arranging for the care of children etc.?
- Did she leave a suicide note?

B. Seriousness of the attempt

- What method was used?
- Did the person understand the consequences of the method she used?:
    a. For example, was the person taking an overdose aware of the actions of the drug and did she believe that the dose taken would be fatal?
    b. Did she take all the tablets or did she leave behind a few?
    c. What are the problems experienced by the patient currently?

(Please see point 10 in step 1)

Step 3: Explore depressive symptoms (see chapter on assessing depression) and/or psychotic symptoms with duration and their impact on current functioning

Step 4: Assess current mental state: mood and hopelessness

- 'How do you feel in yourself?'
- 'How do you see the future?'
- 'Do you still feel that life is not worth living?'

Suicidal thoughts and plans

- 'Do you still have thoughts of harming yourself in any way?'
- 'What do you think you might do?'
- 'Have you made any plans?'
- 'When are you intending to do it?'
- 'What prevents you from doing it?'

Step 5: Past history and background information

- Does she have a past history of suicidal behaviour?
- Does she suffer from a mental illness, for example depression, psychosis, anxiety disorder, borderline personality disorder?
- Is there a history of non-compliance with treatment?
- Does she abuse alcohol or drugs?
- Is there a family history of mental illness, alcohol or substance abuse, violence or suicidal behaviour?

Step 6: Coping methods and ability to seek help

- What were her reactions to previous stresses, failures and losses?
- What does she usually do when there is a problem?
- How does she usually cope?
- With whom does she share her worries?
- How supportive are her family and friends?
- Does she get any help?
- In the past, did anyone offer her any help? How did she find it?

Decision making and developing a management plan

By the end of the assessment, you should be able to answer the following questions, which might help in decision making and formulating a safe management plan:

a. Is there evidence of mental illness?

b. Is there ongoing suicidal intent?

c. Are there non-mental health issues that can be addressed?

d. Ascertain the level of social support available.

Decision making

Following the assessment:

1. If she does appear to have a mental illness, which is of the nature and degree that requires hospital treatment or if she is likely to be at risk to herself should she leave hospital at this time, then try to encourage a voluntary admission. This may help to assess the seriousness of the underlying mental health condition or to allow for a period of inpatient assessment of mental state.

at does not work, it would be appropriate to detain her under
on 5 (2) of the Mental Health Act (doctor's holding power) and
should also let the RMO know that the patient is on Section 5 (2),
hat a Mental Health Act assessment can be arranged as soon as
ible and detention under Section 2 for assessment or Section 3 for
treatment can be considered if necessary.

Developing a management plan

The management plan should be tailored according to the needs of individual patients and it is important to develop a clear plan to help the individual get safely through this period of distress.

The general suggestions for this management plan are outlined below:

- Ensure appropriate supervision/hospitalization for the individual. Immediately after the suicidal attempt, do not leave the individual alone for any length of time. Remove all means of committing suicide.

- If the patient is to be admitted to the hospital, increase the level of nursing observation.

- If the patient is to be discharged from the hospital, involve family members in caring for the individual. Family and friends may be able to provide suitable supervision. Encourage a supportive network away from the clinician (e.g. family, friends, and agencies).

- Ensure the individual has **immediate 24-hour access and support** and consider provision of emergency crisis card giving details of emergency psychiatry service (e.g. crisis team, general practitioner, hospital, telephone support) and telephone contact for emergency counselling or support services. If the individual requires medication, ensure she only has access to a very small amount.

- Neutralize the precipitating problem by encouraging the view that all problems can be solved. Help the individual to resolve any immediate conflicts with others.

- Discuss and agree the management plan with the patient. If the patient is already known to the mental health services, then close liaison with the usual team to agree a joint management plan is very helpful.

- Give a follow-up outpatient appointment with your team in a week's time and make arrangements for one of the members of the community mental health team or the crisis team to contact the patient, within the next 24 hours.

- Engage in Ongoing consultation with superiors or colleagues.

Risk factors for completed suicide

1. Male sex

2. Elderly

3. Single, divorced or widowed

4. Unemployed

5. Living alone with poor social support

6. Previous para suicide or DSH

7. Presence of mental illness/recent history of inpatient psychiatric treatment

8. Concurrent physical illness

9. Recent bereavement

10. History of alcohol and/or drug dependence.

PUERPERAL DISORDER

Task: The A&E staff ask you to see Miss Williams, a young woman who is 2 weeks' postpartum and has presented to the A&E saying 'there is something wrong with her baby boy'. The A&E staff are concerned about her. Take a history and also do a risk assessment.

This station has been asked as a paired/linked station, where in the first station you will be asked to do a risk assessment, and in the next station you may have to discuss with the consultant over the phone about the outcome of your assessment and management plan.

Areas to be concentrated upon

1. Explore the risk factors for postnatal illness

2. Assess bonding and the mother's relationship with her baby

3. Assess the mother's mental state:

   ■ Look for depressive symptoms and negative thoughts such as worthlessness

   ■ Look for psychotic symptoms

   ■ Listen for her thoughts of harming herself and her baby

   ■ Assess her cognitive state and insight.

4. Take a relevant history including past psychiatric history, family history and social support.

Suggested approach

■ Greet the patient and introduce yourself.

■ Explain the purpose of the visit.

■ Obtain permission before you proceed.

■ Use open questions to give the patient an adequate opportunity to ventilate their feelings.

■ The patient may be distressed, paranoid and/or confused and therefore try to acknowledge her distress.

■ Allow her to speak freely, noting her concerns. This may help relieve tension and allow you to assess her mental state.

1. Risk factors

Ask briefly about 4 Ps:

1. Parity
2. Planned/unplanned pregnancy
3. Partner:
   - 'Are you currently in a relationship?'
   - 'How are things between you and your partner/husband?'
   - 'Have there been any difficulties since the baby was born?'
4. Problems during pregnancy and or during labour:
   - 'How did you get on generally during the pregnancy?'
   - 'Tell me about how the delivery went.'

2. Relationship with the baby

- 'Please tell me about your baby.'
- 'How do you feel about your baby?'
- 'How are you coping with the baby?'
- 'Does he sleep well?'
- 'Does he cry too much?'
- 'Have you been losing your temper with the baby?'
- 'Does he have any problems?'

3. Mental state examination

- 'How do you feel in yourself?'
- 'How do you feel as a mother?'
- 'Do you feel useless or worthless as a mother?'
- 'Do you feel trapped as a mother?'
- 'Do you blame yourself for something you have done or thought?'

Ask questions regarding her anxiety about the wellbeing of the baby and any abnormal ideas about the baby:

- 'Are you worried/concerned about the baby?'
- 'Do you have any particular worrying thoughts about the baby? Tell me more about it.'
- 'Do you think there is something wrong with the baby? If so, what do you think is wrong with the baby and why do you think so?'
- 'Are you worried that someone might take the baby away? Who do you think might take the baby away and why would they do so?'

Enquire about depressive symptoms and psychotic symptoms:

- Weepiness, low mood, tiredness, exhaustion
- Anxiety, irritability, insomnia
- Paranoid thoughts, hearing voices or seeing things.

4. Risk assessment – explore any thoughts of her harming herself or the baby

- 'Have you thought of doing something to yourself? If so, what would you do?'
- 'Do you have any thoughts of harming yourself?'
- 'What did you think you might do to yourself?'
- 'Do you feel that you need to do something to the baby?'
- 'Can you explain that please?'
- 'Have you heard voices that tell you to harm the baby?'

5. Relevant history

- Past psychiatric history of depression, bipolar disorder, psychosis, anxiety disorder etc.
- Family history of mental illness, family history of postnatal illness
- Social support – support from friends and family
- Recent significant life stressors
- Any misfortunes like bereavement, the partner's loss of his job, housing, financial problems, etc.

Also assess the cognitive functions and insight at the end of your assessment:

- Cognitive functions – look for disorientation to time and place
- Insight – what do you think is the problem?
- Do you think you might be unwell?

Management

Your management plan should be formulated according to the nature and severity of the postpartum illness. All of the following options should be considered in your management plan, which should be tailored according to the needs of the individual patient:

- Early identification of the presence of postnatal illness

- Education and explanation about the disorder to the patient and the family
- Organize extra support and practical help for the mother either through friends, family or professional help
- Close monitoring of 'those at risk'
- Provide or refer for specific treatments such as individual counselling, marital counselling, and psychotherapy, especially cognitive behavioural therapy
- Depressive episode – appropriate pharmacological intervention with antidepressants
- If depression is severe or associated with thoughts of self-harm or harm to the baby, hospital admission may be required (a specialist mother and baby unit, if possible)
- Psychotic symptoms should be treated with antipsychotic medications and should follow the treatment protocol for treatment of psychotic illness
- For major affective disorders there is also good evidence for ECT and mood stabilizers
- **Prevention** of future episodes through pre-natal education, enhancing coping and stress management techniques such as relaxation training and assertiveness training should be also considered.

Risk factors for postnatal depression

1. Older age
2. Single mother
3. Unplanned pregnancy
4. Personal history of depression
5. Family history of depression
6. Poor social support
7. Significant other psychosocial stressors.

Risk factors for postpartum psychosis

1. Personal history of major psychiatric disorder
2. Previous postpartum psychosis (30% risk of developing psychosis in the subsequent pregnancies)
3. Family history of major psychiatric disorder
4. Single parenthood
5. Lack of adequate social support.

VIOLENCE

Task: Mr White is a 45-year-old man who has a diagnosis of paranoid schizophrenia and has been on long-term antipsychotics. He has a past history of violence to others when unwell and he has recently assaulted a neighbour but was not charged. His CPN has arranged for an assessment with you to assess his current risk of harm to others.

Areas to be concentrated upon

1. Exploration of the violent incident in detail, assess the severity of the violence and the context in which the incident occurred

2. Previous history of violence

3. Current violent impulses and fixed thoughts to harm anybody

4. Explore the current possibility of being acutely psychotic

5. Enquire about compliance with medication and current alcohol and drug use.

Exploration of the incident in detail

- 'Can you describe the incident that happened recently when you lost your control and became violent?'

- 'What caused the incident in the first instance? (Explore the triggers)

- 'Was it just verbal aggression or did you physically hit somebody?'

- 'Did the incident result in injury to others?'

- 'Did you use any weapon during this incident?'

- 'What were you feeling at the time of the violence?'

- 'How do you feel about the whole incident now?' (Explore feelings of guilt/remorse)

Explore whether the patient has a history of violence like hurting others, fights, trouble with the police etc. and also enquire about a family history of violence

- 'Are you the sort of person who has trouble controlling your anger?'

- 'Have you found yourself hitting people when you are angry?'

- 'Have you found yourself damaging property when you are angry?'

- 'What is the most violent thing that you have ever done?'

Current violent thoughts and plans (invite the patient to elaborate further on a positive response)

- 'Is there anything about the present situation that makes you feel like damaging things or hitting people now?'

- 'Do you feel that you might damage things now?'

- 'Do you feel that you might hit people now?'

- 'Are you angry at anyone?'

- 'Who are you angry at?'

- 'Are you thinking about hurting the person mentioned?'

- 'When do you think you might hurt?'

- 'Where will you do this?'

- 'How long have you been thinking this way?'

- 'How do you intend to harm and how serious can it be?'

- 'Do you feel strongly to do so?'

- 'Do you have access to weapons etc?'

- 'Are you able to control these thoughts about hurting?'

- 'Do you think that you would be able to stop yourself from hurting the person if you wanted to?'

Look for psychotic symptoms including threat control-override symptoms

- 'Is there something or someone trying to control you?'

- 'Do you feel under the control of some force or power other than yourself as though you are a robot or a zombie without a will of your own?'

- 'Do you feel that forces beyond your control dominate your mind?'

- 'Are thoughts put in your head that are not your own?'

- 'Do you think that there might be people who intend to do you harm?'

- 'Who are they? What do you intend to do about it?'

- Enquire about command hallucinations and hallucinations of a derogatory or threatening content. (Please check the chapter on eliciting hallucinations.)

- Explore delusions of persecution and reference (Please check the chapter on eliciting delusional ideas.)

- 'Have you been taking your medication regularly?'

- 'Do you think that you might be unwell at the moment?'
- 'In what way do you think you are unwell?'

Substance use (enquire about current alcohol and drug use)

- 'Have you used any alcohol over the past few days?'
- 'Have you used other drugs over the past few days?'
- 'Were you using drugs or alcohol in the past when you were violent?'
- 'Have you taken anything now?'

Note: If the clinician believes that there is real likelihood of violence, then it is important to discuss this with the patient, and it is your duty to inform the concerned people.

The clinician should consider immediate action, which would be to contact the police and warn the individual about the potential risk of violence to him/her.

If in doubt, then seek consultation with a senior colleague.

Potential risk factors for violence

- Being male
- Low intelligence
- Living or growing up in a violent subculture
- Past history of violence
- History of violence in the family
- History of poor impulse control
- Easy access to weapons and victims
- Abuse of drugs or alcohol.

History Taking and
Symptom Elicitation

ALCOHOL HISTORY

Task: Mr Wells, a 43-year-old painter was admitted to the medical ward with acute gastritis. Routine blood tests showed increased GGT and MCV. He gave a history of drinking alcohol almost every day to the medical colleague and therefore the physicians have requested an assessment.

Elicit alcohol history.

Note: Eliciting alcohol history can be asked as a 'paired/linked' station, where in the first station you may be asked to explore the current usage, longitudinal history and to specifically look for features of alcohol dependence.

In the second half of the linked station, you may be asked to discuss the complications suffered following alcohol misuse and also to assess insight and motivation of the patient to stop drinking.

Explore the following:

1. Current usage

2. Longitudinal history

3. CAGE questionnaire

4. Edwards and Gross' criteria for alcohol dependence

5. Risk factors

6. Complications – physical, psychological, social and legal

7. Insight and motivation

8. Rule out mood, psychotic symptoms and or illicit drug abuse.

Note: It would be a good idea to ask at least three or four questions under each subheading and try to obtain a global pass!

Edwards and Gross' criteria for alcohol dependence syndrome

1. Subjective awareness of the compulsion to drink

2. Increased tolerance

3. Withdrawal symptoms

4. Salience of drinking behaviour

5. Reinstatement after abstinence

6. Narrowing of drinking repertoire

7. Relief drinking.

Suggested approach

- Greet the patient and introduce yourself.
- Explain the purpose of the visit.
- Obtain permission before you proceed.
- Build a rapport and address the patient's main concerns first.
- Start with open questions and then proceed to closed questions.

Questions

A. Current usage in a typical day/week

1. 'Do you drink alcohol at all?'
2. 'What do you usually drink?'
3. 'How often do you have a drink?'
4. 'How many drinks do you have on a typical day of drinking?'
5. 'Describe a typical day for me. Could you describe any pattern?'
6. 'What sort of effect does alcohol have on you?'

B. Longitudinal history

1. 'When did it all start?'
2. 'What was the first drink?'
3. 'With whom did you have the first drink?'
4. 'Was it out of your own will (or) peer pressure?'
5. 'How did you progress to the current level?':
   a. Started drinking occasionally (social drink)
   b. Regular weekend drinking.
6. 'How much would you drink at the weekend?':
   a. Regular evening drinking
   b. Regular lunchtime drinking
   c. Early morning drinking (progressive).
7. What did you used to drink in the past and what do you drink now?

C. CAGE questions

- 'Do you feel that you have to **cut** down on your drinking?'

- 'Do people **annoy** you by criticising your drinking?'

- 'Do you feel **guilty** about your drinking?'

- 'Do you have to drink first thing in the **morning** to steady your nerves?'

D. Edwards and Gross' criteria for dependence syndrome

Compulsion

- 'Do you sometimes crave for a drink?' (or)

- 'Do you have a compulsive urge to drink?'

- 'Do you find it hard to stop drinking once you start?'

Tolerance

- 'How much can you drink without feeling drunk? Nowadays, do you need more alcohol to get drunk than you needed before?' (or)

- 'Does a drink have less of an effect on you than before?'

Withdrawal symptoms

- 'What happens if you miss your drink?' (or)

- 'What would happen if you go without a drink for a day or two?' (or)

- 'If you don't drink for a day (or) two, do you experience any withdrawal symptoms such as sweating, shaking, feeling sick, headaches and pounding in your heart?'

Treatment and rapid re-instatement

- Ask about details of treatment and details of any period of abstinence.

- 'What helped you keep off drink?'

- 'Have you ever had an extended period of time when you did not drink?'

- 'What happened to make you start drinking again?'

- 'Have you ever gone to anyone for help with your drink problem?'

- 'Have you ever been in hospital because of your drinking?'

- 'Have you ever been involved in any detoxification programme? Was it completed or not?'

- 'If not, what are the reasons for the failure?'

Primacy

- 'How important is drink compared with other activities for you?'

- 'How often do you miss family and social commitments because of drinking?' (or)
- 'Have you been giving primary importance to alcohol and have you been neglecting other alternative pleasures (or) interests?'

Relief drinking

- 'Do you need a drink first thing in the morning to steady your nerves?'
- 'Do you have to gulp the first few drinks of the day?'

Stereotyped pattern

- 'Do you always drink in the same pub?'
- 'Do you always drink with the same company?'

E. Risk factors for alcohol abuse

Ask about:

- Occupation
- Psychiatric history
- Family history of alcoholism
- Premorbid personality.

Note: As part of the linked station you may be asked to elicit the different types of complications following alcohol misuse and assess insight and motivation.

Physical health problems

'What do you think are the consequences of your drinking?' (open question)

'Have you ever had any health problems due to drinking?'

(Ask specific questions):

- Accidents and head injury
- Memory problems
- Blackouts, falls, fits
- Loss of appetite, weight loss.

Mental health problems

Have you ever had severe shaking, heard voices and seen things that were not there after heavy drinking?

Also ask specifically about:

- Anxiety, depression
- Suicidal ideation/behaviour.

Social problems

Relationship difficulties with the partner, children, family members and friends:

- 'Has your drinking ever led to problems with your family, friends, work or the police?'
- 'How has it affected your family life?'
- 'Have you had any row or arguments with friends or mates?'

Problems at the workplace:

- 'Has your drinking had an effect on your job like missing work, late, Monday absences etc.?'

Financial problems:

- Have you ever had any financial problems because of your habit?

Legal problems (drink driving, drunk and disorderly behaviour, fights while drunk):

- 'Have you actually had an accident or hurt yourself?'
- 'Have you ever been convicted of drink driving?'
- 'Have you ever been arrested because of your drinking?'

Insight and motivation

- 'Do you think that the problems you experience currently are related in any way to your drinking?'
- 'What makes you feel that way and could you please explain that?'
- 'Do you feel you have a problem with alcohol?'
- 'What would you like to do?'
- 'Have you ever thought of giving it up completely?'
- 'What do you think will happen if you give up completely?'

- It is important to rule out mood and psychotic symptoms and also to rule out illicit drug abuse.

- Thank the patient and the examiner.

23

ILLICIT DRUG HISTORY

Task: You are asked to assess this 27-year-old man who has history of using illicit substances such as heroin. Take a detailed history about the usage of illicit substances, looking for features of drug dependence and complications experienced.

Areas to be explored

1. Current usage

2. Longitudinal history

3. Look for features of drug dependence

4. Complications – physical, mental, social and legal

5. Assess insight and motivation

6. Risk assessment – sharing needles, unsafe sex etc.

7. Rule out co-morbidity.

Suggested approach

- Greet the patient and introduce yourself.

- Explain the purpose of the visit.

- Obtain permission before you proceed.

- Build a rapport and address the patient's main concerns first.

- Start with open questions and then proceed to closed questions.

Questions

Open questions

- 'Are there any tablets (or) medicines that you take apart from those you get from your doctor?'

- 'Is there anything that you buy from the chemists (or) get from friends?'

- 'Have you ever used any recreational drugs such as cannabis, cocaine/crack, amphetamines, speed, ecstasy, LSD (or) acid?' (Ask about individual drugs by naming them.)

- 'What about tablets to settle your nerves (or) help you sleep?'

Current usage

- 'What drugs are you using now?'
- 'What is the frequency of use?'
- 'What is the pattern of typical drug use?'
- 'What is the amount of drug taken? (In appropriate measures)'
- 'What effect is the patient seeking when using the drug?'
- 'How much money do you spend in a day/week for getting these drugs?'
- 'What is the route of use? (Oral, smoked, snorted, injected).

  If injected, the following questions are useful to ask:

  a. 'Are needles used?'

  b. 'Where are they obtained?'

  c. 'Are needles shared?'

  d. 'What sites are used for injection?'
- What risky behaviour does the patient engage in?:

  a. 'Injecting and sharing needles'

  b. 'Unsafe sex'

  c. 'Sex for drugs'
- Ask if more than one drug is used at a time
- How is he/she financing the drug use?

Longitudinal history

Ask about the patient's age of first use of drugs, and when the patient started to use the drug regularly

- 'When did you first start to use drugs?'
- 'What was the first drug taken?'
- 'Was it by your own will (or) peer pressure?'
- 'How did you progress to the current level?'
- 'When did you start taking them regularly?'

Features of 'dependence syndrome'

Compulsion

- 'Do you sometimes crave for drugs?'
- 'Do you have a compulsive urge to take drugs?'

Tolerance

- 'Do you have to increase the amount of drugs that you take to get the same effect (or) same amount has given you less effect than earlier?'

Withdrawal symptoms

- 'If you don't take drugs for a day (or 2), do you experience any withdrawal symptoms?' For example, if the patient takes heroin, ask about symptoms such as sweating, gooseflesh, running nose, watery eyes etc.
- Ask the patient to describe them in their own words.

Treatment and re-instatement

Enquire about the patient's past experience of treatment for a drug problem:

- 'Have you ever gone to anyone for help to come out of this?'
- 'Have you ever been in hospital for a drug problem?'
- 'Have there been any periods of abstinence when you were not using any drugs and if so, what has helped you to achieve this?'
- 'What triggers have brought on this habit again?'

Complications

- Have you experienced any complication? (Ask about physical, mental and social complications)
- Have you ever worried about the following?:

    a. Hepatitis B, C and HIV

    b. Complications of injecting like infections, abscesses, sepsis

    c. Accidents, head injury, falls, fits

    d. Anxiety, depression, hearing voices, seeing things

    e. Financial problems

    f. Rows or arguments with friends or family members or in the workplace.

Insight

- 'Do you feel you have a problem with drugs?'
- 'Do you think that the difficulties that you experience currently are related in any way to your drug problems?'

Motivation

- 'What would you like to do?'
- 'Have you ever thought of giving it up completely?'
- 'What do you think will happen if you give up completely?'

■ It is important to rule out mood and psychotic symptoms and also to rule out alcohol misuse.

■ Thank the patient and the examiner.

EATING DISORDER HISTORY

Task: You are asked to see Ms Brown, a 21-year-old bank clerk who has insulin-dependent diabetes mellitus. The GP was concerned about her diabetic control and the patient admitted to omitting her insulin to lose weight. You are asked to elicit an eating disorder history with a view to exploring the psychological issues and abnormal eating pattern.

Explore the following:

1. Psychological issues

2. Eating issues

3. Physical issues

4. Psychosocial stressors

5. Rule out co-morbidity.

Anorexia nervosa

- Weight loss >15% and below expected BMI (body mass index) of 17.5 or less

- Body image distortion – fear of fatness held as an intrusive overvalued idea

- Avoidance of fattening foods, with behaviours aimed at losing weight like vomiting, purging, overexercise, use of appetite suppressants and/or diuretics

- Amenorrhoea in women, a loss of sexual interest and potency in men

- Pubertal delay, if onset is early.

Bulimia nervosa

- Persistent preoccupation with food and eating, and an irresistible craving for food

- Binges – episodes of overeating

- Attempts to counteract the 'fattening' effects of foods by one or more of the following: self-induced vomiting, alternating periods of starvation, purgative abuse, overexercise and use of appetite suppressants, diuretics

- Morbid fear of fatness with imposed 'low weight threshold'.

Suggested approach

- Greet the patient and introduce yourself.
- Explain the purpose of the visit.
- Build a rapport and address the patient's main concerns first.
- Start with open questions and then proceed to closed questions.
- Listen to the patient. Pick up clues from what the patient says to you.

1. Psychological issues

- 'Do you think you have a problem with your weight and eating?'
- 'How do you feel about your weight right now?'
- 'What is your ideal weight?'
- 'Why is that weight ideal for you?'
- 'Are you satisfied with how you look?'
- 'Do you feel fat?/Do you feel ugly?'
- 'How do you feel when you see your image in a mirror?'
- 'Do you feel that you have a distorted body image? If so, in what way?'
- 'Do you fear loss of control? What do you mean by that?'
- 'What do you feel would happen if you did not control your weight (or) eating?'

2. Eating issues

- 'What is a typical day's eating for you?'
- 'Is there a pattern? Does it vary?'
- 'Do you avoid any particular foods? And if so, why?'
- 'Do you restrict fluids?'

Binge eating

- 'Do you ever have times where you feel that your eating is out of control or seems excessive?'
- 'Do you ever binge eat? (i.e. eat during a short space of time, quantities of food that are definitely larger than most people would eat during a similar time and in similar circumstances).'
- 'When did you first start binge eating?'
- 'How often do you do it and why do you do it?'

- 'Could you please describe to me a typical binge?'

Obtain information about type of foods eaten, quantity of food, and duration of the binge:

- 'How do you feel just before you binge?'
- 'Can you identify any particular cause (e.g. feelings, stressors, social situations, etc.) that may trigger the binge?'
- 'How do you feel while you are binge eating?'
- 'How do you feel after bingeing?'

Vomiting

- 'Have you ever had to make yourself sick? If so how?'
- 'How often do you do this?'
- 'Can you tell me why you make yourself vomit?'

Laxatives, diuretics, emetics, appetite suppressants, exercise

- Often many people with these problems use other methods to control their weight like (give examples and ask specifically) taking laxatives, water pills, emetics, and appetite suppressants.
- 'For what reason do you use it?'
- 'Do you fast for a day or more?'
- 'Do you exercise?'
- 'How often do you exercise?'
- 'Is this to burn off calories?'
- 'Do you use exercise as a means of controlling your weight?'

3. Physical symptoms

- Menstrual changes:

  a. 'When was your last period? Are you menstruating regularly?'

- Changes in libido
- Symptoms of anemia: weakness, lethargy, constipation:

  a. 'Do you feel the cold badly?'

  b. 'Have you noticed any weakness in your muscles?'

  c. 'Have you fainted or had dizzy spells?'

4. Explore the possibility of any recent psychosocial stressors

a. Any difficult situation at home or at work

b. Current relationships and any difficulties with it

c. Social activities and life in general

d. Any other recent stressors/stressful life events.

Rule out co-morbidity

- Do not forget to rule out depression and other neurotic symptoms. You can use the same questions in the chapter on depression and anxiety.

- Thank the patient and the examiner.

SYMPTOMS OF DEPRESSION

Task: Mr Jones presented to the A&E department with low mood and sleep disturbance. Do a diagnostic assessment and elicit the symptoms of depression.

Areas to be covered

- Core symptoms of depression
- Biological symptoms
- Cognitive and emotional symptoms
- Ideas of guilt and unworthiness
- Depressive cognition (negative thoughts) and suicidal ideation
- Rule out co-morbidity.

Clinical features suggestive of depression

- Core symptoms – low mood, anhedonia, reduced energy and decreased activity
- Biological symptoms – sleep disturbance, diurnal variation of mood, loss of appetite, loss of weight, loss of libido
- Cognitive symptoms – reduced concentration, poor memory
- Emotional symptoms – reduced self-esteem and low self-confidence
- Ideas of guilt
- Depressive cognitions such as hopelessness, helplessness, worthlessness and suicidal ideation.

Suggested approach

- Greet the patient and introduce yourself.
- Explain the purpose of the visit.
- Build a rapport and address the patient's main concerns.
- Start with open questions and then proceed to closed questions.
- Listen to the patient. Pick up clues from what the patient says to you.

Questions

A. Eliciting core symptoms of depression

Low mood
- 'How are you feeling in yourself?'

- 'How has your mood been lately?'
- 'How bad has it been? Have you cried at all?'
- 'If I were to ask you to rate your mood, on a scale of "1" to "10", where 10 is normal and 1 is as depressed as you have ever felt, how would you rate your mood now?'

Anhedonia

- 'Can you still enjoy the things you used to enjoy?' (or)
- 'Have you lost enjoyment in things you used to enjoy?'
- 'Is the level of enjoyment the same as before?'
- 'What are the things that you find enjoyable/interesting?'

Reduced energy level and decreased activity

- 'How have you been in your energy levels these days?'
- 'Have you been feeling drained of energy lately?'
- 'How do you spend your day?'
- 'Have you wanted to stay away from other people?'

Eliciting biological symptoms

- 'How has your sleep been recently?'
- 'Do you need less sleep than usual?'
- 'Have you had any trouble getting off to sleep?'
- 'Do you wake early in the morning?'
- 'Does you mood vary over the course of the day?'
- 'Is your depression/mood worse at any particular time of day?'
- 'What is the best time/worst time of the day for you?'
- 'What has your appetite been like recently?'
- 'Have you lost any weight lately?'
- 'Has there been any change in your interest in sex?'

Cognitive symptoms

- 'How has your concentration been lately?'
- 'What is your memory like at the moment?'

Emotional symptoms

- 'How confident do you feel in yourself?'
- 'How would you describe your self-esteem?'

Ideas of guilt

- 'Do you feel that you've done something wrong?'
- 'Do you feel guilty about anything at the moment?'
- 'Do you tend to blame yourself at all?'
- 'Do you tend to blame anyone else for your problems?'
- 'Do you have any regrets?'
- 'Do you feel that you've committed a crime, (or) sinned greatly (or) deserve punishment?'

Eliciting suicidal intent and negative thoughts

- 'Do you have any worries on your mind at the moment?'
- 'Have you ever felt that life wasn't worth living?'
- 'How do you see the future?'
- 'Do you feel inferior to others (or) even worthless?'
- 'Do you feel hopeless about yourself?' (or) 'Has life seemed quite hopeless?'
- 'Do you feel helpless?'
- 'Do you feel that life is a burden?'
- 'Do you wish yourself dead?' 'Why do you feel this way?'
- 'Have you had thoughts of ending your life?'
- 'Have you thought about how you would do it?'
- 'Did you actually try?'
- 'Would you do anything to harm yourself or to hurt yourself?'
- 'Have you got any plans to end your life?' 'What plans?'

If the patient says 'yes' to suicidal thoughts, enquire about the frequency of these thoughts; ascertain whether they are only **fleeting** or if it is more **prolonged**. Also check if they are becoming more common.

Duration, course, effects, coping

- 'How long have you been feeling this way?'
- 'What do you think might have caused this?'
- 'How is it affecting your life?'
- 'How do you manage to cope?'

- 'Do you get any help?'

Rule out co-morbidity

1. Anxiety, obsessions

2. Psychosis/hypomania or mania

3. Coping strategies like alcohol and illicit drug use.

■ Thank the patient and the examiner.

HALLUCINATIONS

Task: Mr Smith presented himself to the A&E department in a confused state and complaining of hearing voices. You are asked to assess him and elicit different types of hallucinations.

Areas to cover

- Explore the hallucinatory experience (auditory hallucinations)
- To clarify whether these are elementary/complex hallucinations
- To identify if they are true/pseudo hallucinations
- To clarify whether they are second- or third-person hallucinations
- Explore hallucinations in other modalities
- Duration, effects and coping.

Suggested approach

- Greet the patient and introduce yourself.
- Explain the purpose of the visit.
- Obtain permission before you proceed.
- Build a rapport and address the patient's main concerns.
- Start with open questions and then proceed to closed questions.
- Listen to the patient. Pick up clues from what the patient says to you.

Auditory hallucinations

'I understand that recently you have been hearing voices when there is no one around you and nothing else to explain it. Can you tell me more about it?'

(or) 'I should like to ask you a routine question, which we ask of everybody. Do you ever seem to hear voices (or noises) when there is no one about and nothing else to explain it?'

If the patient agrees, then this experience should be further clarified.

Elementary hallucinations

- 'Do you hear noises like tapping or music?'
- 'What is it like?'

- 'Does it sound like muttering or whispering?'
- 'Can you make out the words?'

Second-person auditory hallucinations

- 'Do you hear voices?'
- 'Can you please give me some examples of the sort of things the voices say?'
- 'Who is it you are talking to? Can you recognize those voices?'
- 'If you recognize them, then whose voices are they?'
- 'How many voices do you hear?'
- 'Do the voices belong to men, women or children?'
- 'Do they speak directly to you?'
- 'Do you hear your name being called?'
- 'Do they tell you what to do? Can you please give me an example?'
- 'Do they give orders? Do you obey?'
- 'Can you carry on two-way conversion with the voices?'

Third-person hallucinations

- 'Do you hear several voices talking about you?' (or)
- 'Do they refer to you as 'he' or 'she' like a third person?'
- 'What do they say?'
- 'Do you hear voices like a running commentary instructing you to do things?'
- 'Do they seem to comment on what you are thinking, reading or doing?'

Confirm whether they are true hallucinations

- 'Where do these voices appear to come from?'
- 'Do you hear them in your mind or in your ears?'
- 'Do the voices come from inside (or) outside your head?'
- 'Do you hear them as clearly as you hear me?'
- 'Can you start or stop them?'
- 'Do you feel that they are real or do you feel that they are just voices?'

Hypnagogic/hypnapompic hallucination

- 'When did this occur? Were you fully awake when you heard these voices?'

- 'Do these voices disturb your sleep?'

- 'Do you hear them more at any particular time like when you go to bed or when you wake up?'

Visual hallucination

- 'Have you seen things that other people can't see?'

- 'What did you see? Can you please give me an example?'

- 'When do you see them and how often?'

- 'Was the vision seen with your eyes (or) in your mind?'

- 'How do you explain it?'

- 'Were you half asleep at that time?'

- 'Has it occurred when you are fully awake?'

- 'Did you realize that you are fully awake?'

Olfactory hallucination

- 'Is there anything unusual about the way things feel or taste or smell?' (open question)

- 'Do you ever notice strange smells that other people aren't bothered by?'

- 'What did you smell? Can you please give me an example?'

- 'How do you explain it?'

Gustatory hallucination

- 'Have you noticed that food or drink seems to have an unusual taste recently?'

- 'What did you taste? Can you please give me an example?'

- 'How do you explain it?'

Tactile hallucination

- 'Have you had any strange or unusual feelings in your body?'

- 'Do you ever feel that someone is touching you, but when you look there is nobody there?'

- 'Some people have funny sensations on the body, for example, insects crawling or electricity passing or muscles being stretched or squeezed. Have you had any such experiences?'
- 'How do you explain it?'

Duration, course, effects, coping

- 'How long have you had these experiences for?'
- 'How often do you have them?'
- 'What do you think might have caused this?'
- 'Why do you think they are happening to you?'
- 'How is it affecting your life?'
- 'How do you manage to cope?'
- 'Do you get any help?'

Rule out co-morbidity

1. Contributing factors to illness and stressors
2. Anxiety
3. Depression
4. Mania/hypomania
5. Coping strategies like alcohol and illicit drug use.

- Thank the patient and the examiner.

FIRST-RANK SYMPTOMS

Task: Mr Brown was referred by his GP complaining of hearing voices and being controlled by some evil forces. Elicit the first-rank symptoms.

Areas to be explored

- Auditory hallucinations – third-person auditory hallucinations, running commentary hallucinations

- Thought–alienation phenomena – thought withdrawal, thought insertion and thought broadcasting

- Passivity phenomena – made feelings, made impulses and made volition or acts, somatic passivity

- Delusional perception

- Clarification, effects and coping.

Schneider's first-rank symptoms are:

Auditory hallucinations:

- Voices heard arguing

- Thought echo

- Running commentary

Delusions of thought interference:

- Thought withdrawal

- Thought insertion

- Thought broadcasting

Delusions of control:

- Passivity of affect

- Passivity of impulse

- Passivity of volitions

- Somatic passivity

Delusional perception.

Suggested approach

- Greet the patient and introduce yourself.

- Explain the purpose of the visit.

- Build a rapport and address the patient's main concerns.

- Start with open questions and then proceed to closed questions.

- Listen to the patient. Pick up clues from what the patient says to you.

'I gather that you have been through a lot of stress and strain recently. When under stress sometimes people have certain unusual experiences. By unusual experience, I mean for example, hearing noises or voices when there was no one about to explain it. Have you had any such experiences?'

If the patient agrees, then this experience should be further clarified:

- 'Can you tell me more about the voices?'

- 'Can you please give me some examples of the sort of things the voice said?'

Third-person auditory hallucinations

- 'Do the voices discuss you between themselves?'

- 'Do you hear several voices talking about you?'

- 'Do they refer to you as "he" (or) "she" as a third person?'

- 'What do they say?'

Running commentary hallucinations

- 'Do you hear voices commenting on what you are doing?'

- 'Do the voices seem to comment on what you are thinking, reading or doing etc?'

- 'Do you hear voices like a running commentary instructing you to do things?'

Hearing thoughts spoken aloud

- 'Are the voices repeating your own thoughts back to you?'

- 'Can you hear what you are thinking?'

- 'Do you ever seem to hear your own thoughts echoed or repeated?'

- 'What is it like?'

- 'How do you explain it?'

- 'Where does it come from?'

Thought alienation phenomenon (open question)

- 'Are you able to think clearly?'

- 'Do you ever get the feeling that someone is interfering with your thoughts? If so, in what way? Could you please explain it?'

Thought broadcasting

- 'Do you feel that your thoughts are private (or) are they accessible to others in any way?'

- 'Can other people read your mind?'

- 'Are your thoughts broadcast, so that other people know what you are thinking?'

- 'How do you know?'

- 'How do you explain it?'

Thought insertion

- 'Are thoughts put into your head that you know are not your own?'

- 'How do you know they are not your own?'

- 'Where do they come from?'

Thought withdrawal

- 'Do your thoughts ever seem to be taken from your head, as though some external person (or) forces were removing them?' (or)

- 'Do your thoughts disappear (or) seem to be taken out of your head?'

- 'Could someone take your thoughts out of your head? Would that leave your mind empty or blank?'

- 'Can you give an example?'

- 'How do you explain it?'

Passivity of affect, impulses and volitions

- 'Are you always in control of what you feel and do?' (Open question)

- 'Is there something or someone trying to control you? What is it?'

- 'Do you feel in control of your thoughts, actions and will?' (or)

- 'Do you ever get the feeling that you are being controlled? That someone else is forcing your thoughts, moods or actions on you?'

- 'Do you feel under the control of some force or power other than yourself as though you are a robot or a zombie without a will of your own?'

- 'Does this force make your movements for you without you willing it?'

- 'Does this force or power impose its feelings on to you against your will?'

- 'Does this force have any other influence on your body?'

Somatic passivity

- 'Does any force possess you?'

- 'What does that feel like?'

- 'Do you feel that someone or some force plays on your body and produces strange bodily sensations like special waves affecting your body?'

- 'Does this force have any other influence on your body?'

- 'Can you please give me an example and can you also describe it for me?'

Delusion perception

- 'Did you at any time realize that things happening around you have a special meaning for you? Can you give me an example?'

- 'Can you explain that? What happened exactly?'

- 'Has a sudden explanation occurred out of the blue to you?'

Clarification, effects and coping

- 'What do you think is causing these experiences?'

- 'How long have you had these experiences?'

- 'Who do you think is causing them?'

- 'Why do they do so? And how do they do that?'

- 'How would you explain them?'

- 'Could it be your imagination?'

- 'How do they affect you? How do they make you feel?'

- 'How would you cope with them? What do you intent to do about them?'

- ■ Thank the patient and the examiner.

DELUSIONS AND OTHER EXPERIENCES

Task: You are seeing Mr Atkins, a 49-year-old postal worker brought to the A&E department by the police. He presented to the police station earlier today, stating that he could no longer hide from the police and he was 'giving himself up'. Explore his thought content and explore his delusional beliefs.

Areas to be covered

- Address the patient's main concerns and the reasons for the presentation.

- Elicit the main abnormal belief and the content of the delusional idea.

- Encourage elaboration and seek explanation of delusional beliefs.

- Assess their onset (primary/secondary) and their fixity (partial/complete).

- Assess the degree of conviction.

- Evaluate effects and coping.

- Screen the patient for the presence of other kinds of delusional beliefs than the one described above.

- Carry out a risk assessment, especially risk of harm to himself or others secondary to the current delusional ideas.

Suggested approach

- Greet the patient and introduce yourself.

- Explain the purpose of the visit.

- Obtain permission before you proceed.

- Build a rapport and address the patient's main concerns.

In this station, explore why he went to the police station today and said that he was 'giving himself up' and what has been worrying him/bothering him. Listen to the patient. Pick up clues from what the patient says to you.

Open questions

- 'Have you experienced anything strange, bizarre or unusual? Or perhaps something that has puzzled you?'

- 'Do you have any particular worries preying on your mind at the moment?'

Delusions of persecution

- 'How well have you been getting on with people?'
- 'Do you ever feel uncomfortable as if people are watching you? (or) talking about you behind your back? (or) paying attention to what you are doing?'
- 'Do you ever feel that people are trying to harm you in any way?'
- 'Is anyone trying to interfere with you or make your life miserable?'
- 'Is anyone deliberately trying to poison you (or) to kill you?'
- 'Is there any organisation like the Mafia behind it?'

Delusions of reference

- 'Do people seem to drop hints about you or say things with a special meaning?'
- 'When you watch television, hear radio or read newspapers, do you ever feel that the stories refer to you directly?' (or)
- 'Do you see any messages for yourself/reference to yourself on TV or radio or in the newspapers?'
- 'When you watch television, hear radio or read newspapers, do you ever feel that the stories refer to things that you have been doing?'

Delusions of control or passivity

- 'Is there anyone trying to control you?'
- 'Do you feel that you are under the control of a person or force other than yourself?'
- 'Do you feel as if you're a robot or zombie with no will of your own?'
- 'Do they force you to think, say or do things?'
- 'Do they change the way you feel in yourself?'

Delusions of grandiosity

- 'How do you see yourself compared to others?'
- 'Is there something "out of the ordinary" about you?'
- 'Do you have any special power or abilities?'
- 'Are you specially chosen in any way?'
- 'Is there a special mission to your life?'

- 'Are you a prominent person (or) related to someone prominent like royalty?'
- 'Are you very rich (or) famous?'
- 'What about special plans?'

Delusions of guilt

- 'Do you feel that you are to blame for anything and that you are responsible for anything going wrong?'
- 'Do you have any regrets?'
- 'Do you have guilt feelings as if you have committed a crime or a sin?'
- 'Do you feel you deserve punishment?'

Nihilistic delusions

- 'How do you see the future?'
- 'Do you feel something terrible has happened or will happen to you?'
- 'Do you feel that you have died?'
- 'Has part of your body died or been removed?' Inquire about being doomed, being a pauper, intestines being blocked etc.

Religious delusions

- 'Are you especially close to God or Christ?'
- 'Can God communicate with you?'

Hypochondriacal delusions

- 'How is your health?'
- 'Do you worry that there is anything wrong with your body?'
- 'Are you concerned that you might have a serious illness?'

Delusions of jealousy

- 'Can you tell me about your relationship?'
- 'Do you feel that your partner reciprocates your loyalty?'

Note:

- If the patient says 'yes' to any of the delusions, then pick up the clues from what the patient says to you.

- Invite the patient to elaborate further on a positive response. Always probe for further elaboration of the beliefs and seek examples.

- Always try to assess the degree of conviction, explanation, effects and coping.

- Also try to assess their onset (primary/secondary) and their fixity (partial/complete).

Conviction, explanation, effects, coping

- What do you think is causing these experiences?

- Who do you think is causing them?

- Why do they do so? And how do they do that?

- How would you explain them?

- Ask how the patient copes with these thoughts, what he/she has done and what he/she intends to do about them.

Always check whether the delusion is:

Primary or secondary
- 'How did it come into your mind that this was the explanation?'

- 'Did it happen suddenly or out of the blue? How did it begin?'

Degree of conviction

- 'Even when you seemed to be most convinced, do you really feel in the back of your mind that it might well not be true, that it might be your imagination?' (or)

- 'Do you ever worry that all of this may be due to your mind playing tricks?'

- Thank the patient and the examiner.

MANIC SYMPTOMS

Task: Miss Brown is a 25-year-old woman who was admitted to the ward with elated mood, hyperactivity and lots of unrealistic active plans for the future. Elicit symptoms of mania.

Areas to be covered

- Core symptoms of hypomania/mania
- Biological and cognitive symptoms
- Overoptimistic ideation and grandiosity
- Exploring grandiose delusions and clarification
- Risk assessment
- Rule out co-morbidity.

Suggested approach

- Greet the patient and introduce yourself.
- Explain the purpose of the visit.
- Obtain permission before you proceed.
- Build a rapport and address the patient's main concerns.
- Start with open questions and then proceed to closed questions.
- Listen to the patient. Pick up clues from what the patient says to you.

Clinical features of mania

- Elevated mood/irritable mood
- Increased energy, which may manifest as overactivity, excitement, reduced need for sleep, pressured speech, racing thoughts and flight of ideas
- Increased self-esteem, evident as overoptimistic ideation, overfamiliarity and grandiosity
- Reduced attention and increased distractibility
- Tendency to engage in behaviour that could have serious consequences such as spending recklessly, sexual disinhibition leading to possible exploitation and reckless driving etc.
- Marked disruption to family life, social activities and occupation.

Questions

Core features of hypomanic/manic symptoms

- 'How are you feeling in yourself?'

- 'Have you sometimes felt unusually/particularly cheerful and on top of the world, without any reason?'

- 'If I were to ask you to rate your mood, on a scale of "1" to "10", how would you rate your mood now?'

- 'Have you felt so irritable recently that you shouted at people or started fights or arguments?'

- 'How is your energy level?'

- 'Do you find yourself extremely active but not getting tired?'

- 'Have you felt particularly full of energy lately (or) full of exciting ideas?'

- 'Have you felt that you were much more active or did many more things than usual?'

Biological symptoms

- 'How are you sleeping?'

- 'Do you need less sleep than usual and found you did not really miss it?'

- 'What has your appetite been like recently?'

- 'Have you lost/gained any weight?'

- 'How is the sexual side of your relationship?'

- 'Have you been more interested in sex recently than usual?'

Cognitive symptoms

- 'What has your concentration been like recently?'

- 'What is your thinking like at the moment?'

- 'Are you able to think clearly?'

- 'Do your thoughts drift off so that you do not take things in?'

- 'Do you find that many thoughts race through your mind and you could not slow your mind down?'

Eliciting overoptimistic ideation and grandiose ideas

- 'How confident do you feel in yourself?'

- 'Do you feel much more self-confident than usual?'
- 'How would you describe your self-esteem to be?'
- 'How do you see yourself compared to others?'
- 'Are you specially chosen in any way?'
- 'Do you have any special powers or abilities quite out of the ordinary? Do you have any special gifts or talents? If so, what are they?'
- 'Is there a special mission to your life?'
- 'Are you a prominent person (or) related to someone prominent like the royalty?'
- 'Are you very rich (or) famous?'
- 'Have you felt especially healthy?'
- 'Have you developed new interests lately?'
- 'Have you been buying interesting things recently?'
- 'Tell me about your plans for the future? Do you have any special plans?'

Clarification, effects and coping

- If the patient harbors grandiose delusions, then pick up the clues from what the patient says to you.
- Invite the patient to elaborate further on a positive response. Always probe for further elaboration of the beliefs and seek examples.
- Always try to assess the degree of conviction, explanation, effects and coping.

Tendency to engage in behaviour that could have serious consequences

- 'Has there ever been a period of time when you were not your usual self and you did things that were unusual for you like spending too much money that got you into trouble?'
- 'Has there ever been a period of time when you were not your usual self and that other people might have thought were excessive, foolish or risky? Can you please give me an example?'

Explore in detail about the symptom history, mode of onset, duration, progress, precipitating factor and associated problems.

Duration, course, effects, coping

- 'How long have you been feeling this way?'

- 'What do you think might have caused this?'
- 'How is it affecting your life?'
- 'How do you manage to cope?'
- 'Do you get any help?'

Rule out co-morbidity such as

- Depression
- Psychotic symptoms
- Coping mechanisms, i.e. drug and alcohol misuse.

■ **Thank the patient and the examiner.**

ANXIETY SYMPTOMS

Task: Mrs Brown is a 41-year-old woman who has been referred to you by her GP to the outpatient clinic for feeling anxious, edgy all the time and fears of 'going crazy'. Elicit a detailed history.

Symptoms of generalized anxiety

- Psychological arousal – fearful anticipation, worrying thoughts, restlessness, poor concentration, irritability, sleep disturbances

- Autonomic arousal – dry mouth, difficulty in swallowing, constriction in the chest, difficulty in breathing, palpitations, chest pain, tremor, headaches, muscle tension, sweating and tingling in the extremities

- Sleep disturbance – insomnia, night terror

- Avoidance of places, situations and people as part of coping strategy.

Areas to cover

- Psychological symptoms of anxiety

- Physical symptoms of anxiety

- Sleep disturbance

- Avoidance mechanism

- Enquire about panic attacks

- Rule out agoraphobias and other phobias

- Rule out co-morbidity.

Suggested approach

- Greet the patient and introduce yourself.

- Explain the purpose of the visit.

- Build a rapport and address the patient's main concerns.

- Start with open questions and then proceed to closed questions given below.

Questions

Eliciting anxiety symptoms

- 'Have there been times when you have been very anxious (or) frightened? What was this like?'

- 'Have you had the feeling that something terrible might happen?'
- 'Have you had the feeling that you are always on the edge?'
- 'Do you worry a lot about simple things?'
- 'Tell me what made you feel so anxious, and tell me about your anxiety symptoms?'
- 'How long have you been feeling so anxious?'
- 'How does it interfere with your life and activities?'
- 'Tell me about your sleep recently. (Explore for sleep disturbance.) Have you had any trouble getting off to sleep?'
- 'Are you sometimes afraid to go to sleep because you know that you will have unpleasant dreams?'
- 'How has your concentration been recently?'
- 'Do you lose your temper more often that you used to?' (Irritability)

Eliciting panic attacks

- 'Have you noticed any changes in your body when you feel anxious?'
- 'Have you had times when you felt shaky, your heart pounded, you felt sweaty, dizzy and you simply had to do something about it?'
- 'Were you getting butterflies in stomach, jelly legs, and trembling of hands?'
- 'Have you ever had a panic attack? What was it like?'
- 'What was happening at the time? Could you please describe it for me?'
- 'How often do you get these attacks?'
- 'How does it interfere with your life and activities?'

Agoraphobia

- 'Do you tend to get anxious in certain situations such as travelling away from home (or) being alone?'
- 'What about meeting people like in a crowded room?'
- 'What about situations like being in a lift or tube?'
- 'Do you tend to avoid any of these situations because you know that you'll get anxious?'
- 'How much does it affect your life?'

Social phobias

- 'Do any particular situations make you more anxious than others?'
- 'Do you tend to get anxious when meeting people, e.g. going into a crowded room and making conversation?'
- 'What about speaking to an audience? What about eating or drinking in front of other people?'

Special phobias

- 'Do you have any special fears like some people are scared of cats or spiders or birds?'

Avoidance

- 'Do you tend to avoid any of these situations because you know that you'll get anxious?'
- 'Do you make any effort to avoid activities, places or people because you know that you will feel more anxious and embarrassed?'
- 'What would you do? How does that make you feel?'

Duration, effects and coping

- 'How long have you been feeling this way?'
- 'What do you think might have caused this?'
- 'How is it affecting your life?'
- 'How do you manage to cope?'
- 'Do you get any help?'

Rule out co-morbidity

- Depression
- Obsessional symptoms
- Anxious personality – 'Would you say you were an anxious person?'

■ Thank the patient and the examiner.

POST TRAUMATIC STRESS DISORDER (PTSD) HISTORY

Task: You have been asked to assess Mr Young, a middle-aged business manager. The patient initially saw his GP because of difficulty in coping with his job. The patient met with an accident 6 months ago. Take a history to establish the features characteristic of the diagnosis of post-traumatic stress disorder (PTSD) and also ascertain the extent of the problem.

Explore the following

1. Ascertain the details of the traumatic incident itself.

2. Look for core features of PTSD that include hyperarousal, intrusions and avoidance.

3. Assess the mode of onset, duration, progression of current symptoms and impairment in different areas of functioning (social and occupational functioning).

4. Rule out co-morbidity.

PTSD

It may begin very soon after the stressful event or after an interval usually of days but occasionally of months, though rarely more than 6 months.

Principal symptoms

Hyperarousal

1. Persistent anxiety and irritability or outbursts of anger

2. Insomnia

3. Poor concentration and exaggerated startle response.

Intrusions

1. Intensive intrusive imagery (flashbacks)

2. Vivid memories

3. Recurrent distressing dreams and nightmares.

Avoidance

1. Actual or preferred avoidance of circumstances resembling, or

2. Emotional detachment and inability to feel emotions

3. Diminished interest in activities.

Others

Inability to recall either partially or completely, some important aspects associated with the stressful event.

Suggested approach

- Greet the patient and introduce yourself.

- Explain the purpose of the visit.

- Obtain permission before you proceed.

- Build a rapport and address the patient's main concerns.

- Start with open questions and then proceed to closed questions.

- Listen to the patient. Pick up clues from what the patient says to you.

I. Traumatic incident

Explore the details of the accident, in particular the perceived severity and establish the level of distress and fear at the time of the event:

- 'Could you describe the accident please?' (Here approach the patient empathetically as it is difficult to talk about traumatic incidents, and acknowledge the patient's distress.)

- Find out about when it happened, how (terrifying) it was?

- Ask about any injuries, in particular head injury, loss of consciousness, whether any other person was injured etc.

- Inquire about any blame, litigation, court cases and their outcome.

2. Core features of PTSD

Intrusions

- 'How often do you think about the accident?'

- 'Do you sometimes feel as if the accident is happening again?'

- 'Do you get flashbacks?'

- 'Have you revisited the scene?'

- 'Do you get any distressing dreams/nightmares of the event?'

- 'What would happen if you hear about an accident?'

- 'Do you have any difficulties remembering parts of the accident?'

Hyper arousal

- 'Have you had the feeling that you are always on the edge?'
- 'Do you tend to worry a lot about things going wrong?' (Feeling anxious)
- 'Do you startle easily?' (Enhanced startle response)
- 'Tell me about your sleep.' (Explore for sleep disturbance)
- 'Are you sometimes afraid to go to sleep?'
- 'How has your concentration been recently?'
- 'How has your memory been lately?'
- 'Do you lose your temper more often that you used to?' (Irritability)

Avoidance

- 'How hard is it for you to talk about the accident?'
- 'Do you deliberately try to avoid thinking about accidents?'
- 'Have you been to the place where the accident happened?'
- 'Do you make any effort to avoid the thoughts or conversations associated with the trauma? How would you do that?'
- 'Do you make any effort to avoid activities, places or people that arouse recollection of the trauma?'

Emotional detachment and numbness

- 'How do you feel in yourself generally?'
- 'Have there been any changes in your feelings generally?' (Emotional detachment).
- 'How do you see the future?'

3. Assess the duration, progress, severity, frequency of current symptom and impairment of normal functioning

'I would like to know how your problems have been affecting you, your family and social life.' (Open question):

- 'How do you feel in yourself generally?'
- 'How has all this been affecting you?'
- 'How do you spend your time these days?'
- Enquire about effect on family, social life and work.

4. Rule out co-morbidity

a. Mood symptoms, especially depression

b. Other anxiety symptoms

c. Current coping mechanisms including drugs and alcohol.

Explore premorbid personality, past history

- Before all this happened, what sort of a person were you?

- How did you cope with stress?

- Have you had any mental health problems before the accident?

■ **Finally it is important to thank the patient and the examiner.**

OBSESSIVE–COMPULSIVE DISORDER SYMPTOMS

Task: Miss Smith is a 27-year-old woman who has come to your clinic following referral by her GP. She mentioned that she is extremely concerned about cleanliness and washes her hands several times a day. Talk to her about her current problems and elicit features of obsessive–compulsive disorder.

Areas to cover

- Obsessional thoughts – ideas, images or impulses

- Compulsive acts/rituals – washing, cleaning, checking, counting

- Resistance and avoidance

- Duration, effects and coping

- Rule out co-morbidity–depression, anxiety.

Suggested approach

- Greet the patient and introduce yourself.

- Explain the purpose of the visit.

- Build a rapport and address the patient's main concerns.

- Start with open questions and then proceed to closed questions.

- Listen to the patient. Pick up clues from what the patient says to you.

'I gather that your doctor has referred you to my clinic today. Can you tell me briefly about what has been bothering you?' (Open question)

Questions

Obsessional thoughts

- 'Do any unpleasant thoughts/ideas keep coming back to your mind, even though you try hard not to have them?' (or)

- 'Do you have any recurring thoughts, ideas, or images that you cannot get rid of in your mind?'

- 'How often do you have these thoughts?'

- 'Are these thoughts your own or are they put into your mind by some external force?'

- 'Where do they come from?'

- 'What is it like? How do you explain it?'

- 'What do you do when you get these thoughts?'

- 'Are they distressing, and if so, in what way?'

- 'Is there anything you try to do to stop these thoughts?'

- 'What happens when you try to stop them?'

Compulsive acts

- 'Do you ever find yourself spending a lot of time doing the same thing over and over again even though you have already done it well enough?' For example:

- 'Do you spend a lot of time on personal cleanliness, like washing over and over even though you know that you're clean?'

- 'Does contamination with germs worry you?'

- 'Do you find that you have to keep on checking things that you know that you have already done?' (like gas taps, doors, and switches)

- 'What happens when you try to stop them?'

- 'Do you have to touch (or) count things many times?'

- 'Do you have any other rituals?'

- 'Do you find it difficult to make decisions even for simple trivial things?' (Obsessional ruminations)

- 'Do you have any impulses to do unwise things?'

- 'What kind of impulses do you have and do you ever give in to these?'

Explore in detail about the symptom history, mode of onset, duration, precipitating factors and associated problems.

Duration, effects and coping

- 'How long have you been feeling this way?'

- 'What do you think might have caused this?'

- 'How is it affecting your life?'

- 'How do you manage to cope?'

- 'Do you get any help?'

Co-morbidity

Ask about associated symptoms, such as:

- Depression, generalized anxiety, phobias
- Anankastic personality traits – 'Do you tend to do/keep things in an organized way?'

■ Thank the patient and the examiner.

ASSESSING INSIGHT

Task: Mr Smith is a 35-year-old man who is curently an informal inpatient with a diagnosis of paranoid schizophrenia. He suffers from prominent auditory hallucinations and has been started on risperidone. He has a past history of non-compliance to treatment and you have been asked to assess his insight.

Insight assessment

■ Believing that their abnormal experiences are symptoms and the symptoms are attributable to psychiatric illness

■ Belief that assistance of some kind is needed to help with the problems

■ Assess attitude to treatment and psychiatric services.

Questions

● 'I understand that recently you have been hearing voices when there is no one around you and nothing else to explain it. Could it be that your experiences are part of an illness affecting your mind?' (or)

● 'You described several symptoms ... namely ... and what is your explanation of these experiences? Do you think that the symptoms were part of your nervous condition?'

● 'Do you consider that you are ill in any way?' (or)

● 'Do you think there is anything the matter with you?'

● 'What do you think it is? Do you have a physical or mental illness?'

● 'Could it be a nervous condition? What is it?'

● 'Do you feel that you need help to deal with this problem?'

● 'What kind of help do you think would be useful?'

● 'Do you need treatment for a mental problem now?'

● 'Why do you think that you have come into the hospital?'

● 'What do you feel about being in hospital?'

● 'Do you think that it has helped you to be here? If so, in what way?'

● 'Has the medication been helpful?'

● 'Do you think that medication helps you to remain well?'

● 'Will you take the recommended medication for the future?'

● 'Have any other treatments been helpful?'

■ Thank the patient and the examiner.

MENTAL STATE EXAMINATION

Task: Mr White presented to the A&E department in a confused state and complained of hearing voices. Carry out a mental state examination for this man.

The Mental State Examination is designed to obtain information about specific aspects of the individual's mental experiences at the time of the interview.

Remember the following order

- Appearance and behaviour
- Speech
- Mood
- Thought
- Perception
- Cognition
- Insight.

Note: There is no need to comment about behaviour and speech in this station unless the examiner specifically asks you. Most candidates generally tend to forget to assess cognitive state and insight, which are also important components of mental state examination, and it carries equal credit in marks as that of mood, thoughts and perception.

Suggested approach

- Greet the patient and introduce yourself.
- Explain the purpose of the visit.
- Obtain permission before you proceed.
- Build a rapport and address the patient's main concerns first.
- It is generally considered to be a good idea to enquire about the patient's mood and then take it from there.

Mood

- 'How are you feeling in yourself?'
- 'How has your mood been lately?'
- 'How bad has it been? Have you cried at all?'

- 'If I were to ask you to rate your mood, on a scale of "1" to "10", where 'ten is normal and one is as depressed as you have ever felt, how would you rate your mood now?

For further questions, please see chapter on 'Eliciting symptoms of depression'.

Thoughts

'Can you think clearly or is there any interference with your thoughts?' (Open question)
When investigating thoughts, also enquire about:

- Obsessions, phobia

- Preoccupations

- Delusional ideas

- Depressed negative thoughts

- Thoughts of self-harm or of harming other people.

Delusions

Explore the different types of delusions that would include delusions of control or passivity, delusions of persecution, delusions of reference, delusions of grandiosity, delusions of thought interference (thought withdrawal, thought insertion, thought broadcasting) and all other types of delusions.
(Please see chapter 'Delusions and other Experiences' for more information.)

Perception

Hallucinations: Check hallucinatory experiences, mainly auditory and visual, but it is also important to check hallucinations in other modalities as well. (Please see chapter 'Eliciting hallucinations' for further information.)
Illusion: Did the vision seem to arise out of a pattern on the wallpaper or a shadow?
Ask about other perceptual disturbances.

Depersonalisation:

- 'Do you ever feel unreal?' (or)

- 'Have you ever felt as if your body or parts of body were unreal or foreign?'

- 'Can you describe it please?'

Derealisation:

- 'Do you ever feel that things around you are unreal?'

- 'Can you describe it please?'

Cognition

Orientation

- Time (day, date, year, time of the day)
- Place (name of the place/hospital/floor)
- Person.

Attention and concentration: Subtracting serials of 7s from 100, Spell W-O-R-L-D backwards.

Memory

- Working memory: Digit span 6 plus or minus 1
- Short-term memory: Name and address: immediate and 5-minute recall
- Long-term memory:

  Personal events:

  a. When did you get married?

  b. When did you finish school?

  General events:

  a. Who is the prime minister of the UK?

  b. Has anything important happened in the world recently?

Insight

- 'Do you think there is anything the matter with you?'
- 'What do you think it is?'
- 'Could it be a nervous condition?'
- 'Do you think that the symptoms were part of your nervous condition?'

- ■ Thank the patient and the examiner.

PREMORBID PERSONALITY

Task: Elicit the premorbid personality of this 42-year-old man who has come to see you in your outpatient clinic. Ideally, collateral history is necessary to elicit premorbid personality.

Areas to be covered

- Screening for paranoid, schizoid, schizotypal personality traits
- Screening for antisocial, borderline and histrionic personality traits
- Screening for anxious, dependent and anankastic personality traits
- Predominant mood
- Interpersonal relationships
- Coping strategies
- Hobbies, interest and beliefs.

Questions

Start with open questions:

- 'How would you describe yourself as a person before you were ill?'
- 'How do you think other people would describe you as a person?'

Then ask closed questions about individual personality traits:

Cluster A (paranoid, schizoid, schizotypal)

- 'How do you get on with people?' (Paranoid)
- 'Do you trust other people?' (Paranoid)
- 'Would you describe yourself as a "loner"?' (Schizoid)
- 'Were you able to make friends?'
- 'Do you have any close friends?' (Schizoid)
- 'Do you indulge in fantasies? Sexual and non-sexual fantasies, daydreaming?'
- 'Do you like to be around other people or do you prefer your own company?'

Cluster B (antisocial, borderline and histrionic)

- 'What's your temper like?' (Antisocial, emotionally unstable)
- 'How do you deal with criticisms?'
- 'Are you an impulsive person?' (Impulsive)
- 'Do you take responsibility for your actions?' (Antisocial, impulsive)
- 'Are you overemotional?' (histrionic)
- 'How do you cope with life?' (Borderline)
- 'How do you react to stress?' (Borderline)
- 'Do you maintain long-term relationships with people?' (Antisocial, borderline)
- 'Do you often feel that you are empty inside?'

Cluster C (anxious, dependent and anankastic)

- 'Are you anxious (or) shy?' (Anxious/avoidant)
- 'Are you a worrier?' (Anxious, dependent)
- 'How much do you depend on others?' (Dependent)
- 'Would you describe yourself as a perfectionist?' (Anankastic)
- 'Do you tend to keep things in an orderly way?' (Anankastic)
- 'Do you have unusually high standards at work/home?' (Anankastic)

Enquire about:

1. Predominant mood

- Optimistic/pessimistic
- Stable/prone to anxiety
- Cheerful/despondent.

2. Interpersonal relationships

- Current friendships and relationships
- Previous relationship – ability to establish and maintain
- Sociability – family, friends, work mates and superiors.

3. Coping strategies

- How does the patient cope with problems?

- 'When you find yourself in difficult situations, what do you do to cope?'

4. Personal interests – hobbies, leisure time

- 'What sort of things do you like to do to relax?'

5. Beliefs – religious beliefs

- 'Are you religious?'

6. Habits – food fads, alcohol, current/previous use of drugs (etc.)

■ Thank the patient and the examiner.

DEMENTIA – OBTAINING COLLATERAL HISTORY

Task: You are in the memory clinic and you have been asked to assess Mr Smith, an 82-year-old man who suffers from memory problems. However, you want to get more information about him from Mrs Smith. Obtain a collateral history from Mrs Smith.

In the exam, you may be asked to take a collateral history about dementia in general or about specific types such as vascular dementia, Lewy body dementia and fronto-temporal dementia. However, the format would remain almost the same and the areas to be covered are outlined below.

Important areas to be covered

- Mode of onset, duration and progression of the symptoms
- Ask in detail about cognitive, behavioural, psychological, physical and biological symptoms
- Risk assessment
- Past medical history
- Past psychiatric history
- Relevant personal history
- Relevant family history.

Note: This can be asked as a 'paired/linked' station, where in the first part you may be asked to obtain collateral history from the patient and in the second part of the linked station, you may be asked to discuss the outcome of your assessments, treatment options and psychogeriatric services available for patients with dementia (please see Alzheimer's disease, p108).

Suggested approach

- Greet the patient and introduce yourself.
- Explain the purpose of the visit.
- Obtain permission before you proceed.
- Address her main concerns.
- Allow her to speak freely for the first few moments, noting her concerns.
- Start with open questions.

- Introduce yourself to the patient's relative and address the main concerns:

  a. 'Please describe for me the problems your husband has been having?' (Open question)

  b. 'Can you give me examples of his forgetfulness?'

  c. 'Is there anything else you are concerned about?'

- Onset and progression:

  a. 'When did the symptoms start?'

  b. 'What symptoms were noticed first?'

  c. 'Did it start gradually or suddenly?'

  d. 'Has it progressed gradually or suddenly?'

  e. 'Are there any fluctuations?'

1. Cognitive symptoms

Inquire about symptoms in all cognitive domains.

Memory (Make sure that you enquire about both short-term and long-term loss, if present)

Short-term memory

Can he remember things that happened in the last few minutes or in the day?:

- 'Can you give me some examples?'

- 'Like forgetting people's names'

- 'Like forgetting appointments or important dates?'

- 'Like forgetting conversations they have had with people'

- 'Like forgetting where they have put things (misplacement of personal and household items)'

- 'Repeating oneself, asking the same question more than once'

- 'Forgetting to take medication or taking it twice etc.'

Long-term memory

- 'Can he remember events that happened a few years ago?'

- 'Can you please give me some examples?'

- 'Does prompting or recognition help?'

- 'Is it consistent or patchy?'

Temporal and spatial disorientation

- 'Does he know the time of the day, the day of the week, date of the month etc?'
- 'How often does he lose his way at home or in the neighbourhood?'
- 'What about getting lost on what are familiar routes?'

Language difficulties

- 'How about the way he speaks?'
- 'Does he have any word-finding problems?'
- 'Can he understand when someone speaks to him?'

Dyspraxia

- 'The memory problems that you describe, do they affect his ability to look after himself, or to do the things he used to?'
- 'Does he have difficulty doing things for himself like maintaining personal hygiene, washing, cooking, laundry etc?' (Activities of daily living)
- 'Has he got difficulty in cooking a meal or organising bills to be paid?' (Activities of daily living)
- 'Is he able to handle money?'
- 'Can he do his own shopping?'

Dyslexia, dysgraphia

- 'What about reading and writing?'

Visuospatial difficulties, agnosia

- 'Does he have difficulty recognising things, places or people?'
- 'Does he have difficulty in recognising familiar faces?'

Judgement, decision making

- 'What about planning, making decisions etc?'
- 'Does he have difficulty in solving everyday problems that he used to solve?'

2. Behavioural symptoms

- 'Has there been any change in his behaviour like being more irritable than usual?'
- 'Have you noticed any change in personality that seems to have occurred recently?'

- Ask about becoming aggressive frequently, episodes of violent and anger outbursts.
- Also enquire about behaving inappropriately, being socially withdrawn, wandering at night-time, disinhibited behaviour, repetitive behaviours etc.

3. Psychological symptoms

- Enquire about symptoms of depression (low mood, crying spells) and anxiety.
- Also enquire about paranoia, auditory and visual hallucinations and other psychotic symptoms.

4. Physical symptoms

Ask briefly about:

- Sensory impairment
- Weakness of limbs
- Gait disturbance
- Parkinson's disease – any abnormal movements
- Incontinence.

5. Biological symptoms

Inquire about:

- Sleep disturbance and symptoms getting worse at night
- Appetite disturbance
- Loss of weight.

Risk assessment

- Fire risk – safety in the home, the cooker used safely, smoking etc.
- Management of finances
- Inappropriate use of medication
- Risk of driving.

Other relevant factors in the patient's history

- Current medication
- Past medical history
  a. High blood pressure
  b. Diabetes

c. Thyroid disorders

d. Infections

e. Stroke

- Past psychiatric history: particularly depression
- Family history of dementia
- Risk factors for dementia

a. Alcohol

b. Head injury

- Personal history

a. Education

b. Occupation

c. Living situation.

■ Thank the relatives for their help.

■ Explain that we need to assess him further and would like to perform some memory tests, blood tests and a brain scan.

Note: The diagnostic criteria for all the common dementias are given below.

Dementia in Alzheimer's disease (diagnostic criteria)

- Global deterioration in intellectual capacity and disturbance in higher cortical functions like memory, thinking, orientation, comprehension, calculation, language, learning abilities and judgement, an appreciable decline in intellectual functioning and some interference with personal activities of daily living
- Insidious onset with slow deterioration
- Absence of clinical evidence or findings from special investigations suggestive of organic brain disease or other systemic abnormalities
- Absence of sudden onset or physical/neurological signs.

Remember 5 As

- Amnesia – impaired ability to learn new information and to recall previously learned information
- Aphasia – problems with language (receptive and expressive)
- Agnosia – failure of recognition, especially people

- Apraxia – inability to carry out purposeful movements even though there is no sensory or motor impairment
- Associated disturbance – behavioural changes, delusions, hallucinations.

Vascular dementia

- Presence of a dementia syndrome, defined by cognitive decline from a previously higher level of functioning and manifested by impairment of memory and of two or more cognitive domains (orientation, attention, language, visuospatial functions, executive functions, motor control and praxis) and deficits should be severe enough to interfere with activities of daily living not due to physical effects of stroke alone.
- Onset may usually follow a cerebrovascular event and is more acute.
- Course is usually stepwise, with periods of intervening stability.
- Focal neurological signs and symptoms or neurological evidence of cerebrovascular disease (CVD) judged etiologically related to the disturbance. CVD defined by the presence of focal signs on neurological examination, such as hemiparesis, lower facial weakness, Babinski sign, sensory deficit, hemianopia and dysarthria and evidence of relevant CVD by brain imaging (CT or MRI).
- Emotional and personality changes are typically early, followed by cognitive deficits that are often fluctuating in severity.
- Symptoms not occurring during the course of the delirium.

Dementia with Lewy bodies

- Spontaneous motor features of Parkinsonism
- Fluctuating cognition with pronounced variation in attention and alertness
- Recurrent visual hallucinations, which are typically well formed and detailed
- Progressive cognitive decline of sufficient magnitude to interfere with normal social and occupational functioning and memory loss may not be an early feature but it is usually evident with progression
- Supportive features: Neuroleptic sensitivity and history of falls.

Lewy body dementia: If both motor symptoms and cognitive symptoms develop within 12 months, then it is conventional to give a diagnosis of Lewy body dementia.

Parkinson's disease dementia: If the Parkinsonian symptoms have existed for more than 12 months before dementia develops then a diagnosis of Parkinson's disease dementia is given.

Frontotemporal dementia

- Insidious onset and gradual progression

- Early loss of personal and social awareness

- Early emotional blunting, early loss of insight

- Behavioural features: Early signs of disinhibition, decline in personal hygiene and grooming, mental rigidity, inflexibility, hyperorality, stereotyped and perseverative behaviour

- Speech disorder: Reduction and stereotypy of speech, echolalia, and perseveration

- Affective symptoms: Anxiety, depression, and frequent mood changes, emotional indifference

- Physical signs: Incontinence, primitive reflexes, akinesia, rigidity and tremor.

Counselling/Explanation About a Particular Disease or Condition

SCHIZOPHRENIA

Task: Mrs Bennett is the divorced mother of one of your patients, Stephen Bennett, who is a 21-year-old university student recovering from a recurrence (second episode) of a schizophrenic illness. This first presented with an acute onset 3 years ago. He stopped medication 1 year after the first episode and relapsed 6 months ago. Both illnesses were of sudden onset and symptoms included auditory hallucinations and thought withdrawal. His mother is very worried. She has asked to discuss him with you at the outpatient clinic. Her son is willing for you to discuss his case with his mother. Explain the nature of schizophrenia and the long-term prospects for her son.

Note: This could be asked as a 'linked/paired' station, where in the first half of the scenario you will be asked to elicit symptoms of schizophrenia, and in the second half of the scenario, you may have to discuss with the patient's relative about this condition.

Suggested approach

- Greet the patient and introduce yourself.
- Explain the purpose of the visit.
- Obtain permission before you proceed.
- Build a rapport and address the relative's main concerns.

What is schizophrenia?

Most people have heard the word 'schizophrenia' but are not really sure what it means. Schizophrenia is a common mental illness, which affects one person in 100. It usually develops in the late teens or early twenties, although it can start in middle age or even much later in life.

It is a mental health condition in which a person finds it difficult to decide what is real and what is not real – it is a bit like having a dream when you are wide awake.

How can it affect an individual?

It can affect an individual's everyday life in many ways, such as:

- A person with schizophrenia may act in an odd or strange way. The person's thinking may be muddled and confused and they may have abnormal experiences.
- They may have trouble handling everyday problems. They may not be able to concentrate or think clearly.

- They may find it hard to make conversation or show feelings, which can make it difficult to get on with people.

- Sometimes the person may stop taking care of their basic needs.

- Symptoms may be described as positive or negative. These are divided into positive symptoms, which are abnormal experiences, and negative symptoms, which indicate decrease or absence of normal behaviour.

What causes schizophrenia?

No one as yet knows for sure what causes it. There seem to be a number of different causes. Schizophrenia is probably caused by a disturbance in the working of the brain, possibly due to chemical imbalance. It is not clear what happens when a person develops schizophrenia, but it is thought that chemicals in the brain are affected, resulting in the symptoms of hallucinations, delusions and difficulty thinking.

It is believed that genetic factors provide about half the explanation for the illness. Sometimes, street drugs like cannabis, cocaine, ecstasy, or amphetamines can bring on this illness. It does seem that smoking cannabis can make matters worse in those who already suffer from schizophrenia.

Since the illness often occurs when the person is under stress, it is thought that stress may act as a trigger.

Can schizophrenia be inherited?

Yes it can. However, this does not mean that if someone in your family has schizophrenia everyone will have it. Nor does it mean that a person with schizophrenia should not marry and have children. It means that if a close relative (e.g. brother, parent or sister) has it, then your chance of getting the illness is higher. Remember that it is not the illness itself that is inherited, but the tendency to get the illness.

Is schizophrenia a split mind?

There is a common idea that it means having more than one personality or a split personality. This is untrue. People with schizophrenia have only one personality, although their personality may be disturbed in some way.

Doesn't schizophrenia make people unpredictable and dangerous?

People who suffer from schizophrenia are rarely dangerous. They are no more unpredictable than anyone else. Despite what is reported in the newspapers people with mental illness and, in particular, schizophrenia are rarely violent but are more likely to be quiet, shy and afraid of what is happening to them.

Street drugs or alcohol usually sparks off any violent behaviour. This is the same as for people who do not suffer from schizophrenia.

Can families cause schizophrenia?

In the past, people believed that disturbed parents and families caused schizophrenia. Research has proven that families cannot, and do not, cause schizophrenia.

However, stressful events, or difficult relationships in the family can sometimes trigger an episode of schizophrenia in someone who is otherwise likely to develop it because of genetic and other factors.

How will I know if my relative has schizophrenia?

There is no specific test for schizophrenia. Doctors diagnose schizophrenia when a person displays a specific group of symptoms. Doctors and psychiatrists find out what symptoms are present, from what the patient and their relatives tell them.

What are positive symptoms?

These are the symptoms that individuals experience such as disturbance of thinking process, delusions and hallucinations:

- Disturbance of thinking can occur in different ways, for example, thoughts being put into your head, which seem to come from other people, by telepathy or radiowaves.

- Thoughts leaving your head as if someone is taking them out, so that your mind is blank and you are unable to think about anything.

- Thoughts seeming to be spoken aloud so that everyone knows what you are thinking and none of your thoughts are private.

What are delusions?

A delusion is a false belief that appears to be quite real to the person with schizophrenia, for example:

- Believing that another person has control of your thoughts or actions, and that you are unable to stop them

- Believing that someone is trying to harm you or kill you for no good reason, or that you are being persecuted

- Believing that things you see or read about have a special message for you

- Believing that you are a special person or that you have some special powers.

What are hallucinations?

Hallucinations are false perceptions. This means that the person hears, sees or smells things that cannot be heard, seen or smelt by others. Hearing voices is a very common symptom of schizophrenia. The voices will appear real to the person and may come from the next room or outside. Sometimes they will seem to come from inside a person's head or from a part of their body or, they believe that something or someone is touching them when there is no one there and nothing to explain this.

What are negative symptoms?

These symptoms are usually apparent as changes in a person's behaviour. They are called negative symptoms because they indicate decreases or absences of normal behaviour. For example:

- Lack of motivation to do anything.

- A decrease in all activity levels – ranging from hobbies and leisure pursuits to self-care such as washing.

- Inability to show any emotion; the person may appear flat and may not show any feelings or emotions.

- Inability to enjoy activities that used to give pleasure.

- Disinterest in conversation and talking; the person will not start conversations and will answer with one word, if at all.

These symptoms can be very distressing for relatives. However, it is important to remember that these symptoms are part of the illness and not due to the person's being lazy or hurtful.

Are there any other symptoms?

Yes, there are other symptoms worth mentioning such as language difficulties, odd habits and changed feelings or emotions:

- **Language difficulties:** Sometimes people with schizophrenia will talk in a way that is hard to follow. They may make up words or use odd expressions.

- **Odd habits:** These may include standing or sitting in unusual ways, peculiar mannerisms or habits.

- **Changed feelings or emotions:** Sometimes people with schizophrenia show no feelings or emotions. At other times they may laugh or cry when they are not feeling happy or sad.

What should I do if I think my relative has schizophrenia?

If you think your relative has schizophrenia then you should encourage the person to see his/her GP. If the person is unwilling or refuses to see the GP then you should contact his/her GP and seek advice.

How do you treat this illness?

When a person becomes mentally ill, they are usually treated in the hospital for a further assessment and diagnosis to be made. Afterwards, they can often be treated whilst living at home, especially if they have a supportive family.

Drugs help to alleviate the most disturbing symptoms of the illness. However, they do not provide a complete answer. Support from families and friends, other forms of treatment and services such as supported housing, day care and employment schemes also play a vital role.

What medications are there and how do they work?

There are medications called 'antipsychotics' that help to reduce the symptoms and the anxiety associated with the symptoms. These are made up of chemicals that alter and correct the chemical imbalance in the brain.

Medication is the mainstay of treatment for schizophrenia. We can't cure the illness completely but we can control the symptoms.

Medication works in two ways:

1. It reduces the symptoms of an attack of the illness.

2. Once the symptoms have improved it helps prevent further attacks or the symptoms getting worse.

What will happen if I stop taking my medication? (if the patient asks this question)

If an individual stops taking his/her medication against the advice of their doctor then the chances of their having an attack of schizophrenia are more than doubled. It is, therefore, very important that an individual keeps taking their medication even when they feel completely well.

Is there any medication that has been proven to work?

All antipsychotic medication has a beneficial effect on the symptoms of schizophrenia, but individual patients respond differently to different medication and may need different doses to have the desired effect.

Does the medication have any side effects?

Yes, unfortunately, medication for the treatment of schizophrenia can have unwanted side effects. These are not usually life threatening, and should be discussed with the doctor or psychiatrist. Some common side effects include drowsiness, shakiness, restlessness, muscle stiffness, increased appetite, weight gain, dry mouth and dizziness, especially when standing up suddenly. The good news is some of the newer medication does not have the unpleasant side effects of restlessness, muscle stiffness, and shakes and is equally effective.

How long will he/she have to continue the medication?

The medication controls the symptoms and promotes recovery, but it does not cure the illness. The symptoms often tend to come back. This is much less likely to happen if the person continues taking medication even when they feel well. For most people, the symptoms usually come back in about 6 months after stopping medication. A small number of people are able to stop medication with no ill effects. Most people, however, need to take maintenance therapy indefinitely, to prevent relapse. For the best outcome, everyone involved, including the person, the family, the community psychiatric team and others need to work together from an early stage.

How effective is treatment? What happens in the long term?

We can't cure schizophrenia. We can only control the symptoms. Some people have only one attack but many people will experience periods when the symptoms return – these are called relapses. A few sufferers will have symptoms all the time.

The illness is likely to affect studies, work and social life. However, many people with schizophrenia live independently, and more and more people are able to work and to have families.

What other treatments would/could be useful?

Several other forms of therapy may be helpful in assisting recovery, in addition to the conventional treatments. Some examples are:

- Talking therapy
- Family therapy
- Relaxation therapy
- Exercise.

How can I help my relative?

Once a person has been diagnosed with schizophrenia the family and the environment in which they live can contribute in a positive or negative way. You can help your relative or friend who is suffering from schizophrenia in a number of ways:

- By encouraging the person to take their medication, especially when they are feeling well.

- By trying to reduce stressful events or helping the person to cope with stress. Major stressful events such as a death in the family, loss of job or break up of a relationship can make schizophrenia worse or trigger off a relapse of symptoms. Where stressful events cannot be avoided, try and give the person as much notice as possible to introduce change in a gradual way. It is impossible to avoid all stress. However, family members can help one another to cope with difficulties.

- People can support the individual by encouraging them to regain their former skills. If they nag or criticise the person or push them too hard, it may make things worse. On the other hand if too much is done for them, this can make them worse too. Try not to be too fussy or overprotective. It is very important that the person is encouraged to lead an independent life and gain confidence.

- Sometimes the person may become depressed and fed up. This is difficult to cope with, but the family members and friends can try to be sympathetic and supportive. Try to build up their confidence and be encouraging and positive.

- Living with a person with schizophrenia can be challenging. They may behave in strange ways; stay in bed all day or take hours to get things done. They may seem as though they don't care about anything or anyone. It is hard not to get angry, but this will not help. Try to be patient and encourage gradual change – try not to criticise or punish the person. Encourage the patient and praise their efforts.

Are there any rehabilitation programmes available?

Schizophrenia makes it difficult to deal with the demands of everyday life. Ordinary activities like washing, answering the door, shopping, or making a phone call can seem like huge hurdles. To some extent, drugs help to overcome such problems. However, it is more helpful in the long run if support includes nurses, key workers, occupational therapists and other members of the community mental health team. These provide access to a wide range of services.

After an acute illness, it is often helpful to attend a day unit, starting with physical activities and going through creative pursuits such as painting and pottery to more demanding 'work-like' activities. The idea is to help people get into or back to work. Other services such as unemployment initiatives, and sheltered work, supported accommodation schemes, drop-in centres and day care facilities also play a vital role. For those people whose illness is more prolonged and severe, a specialist rehabilitation service, including residential care may be available.

What is the community mental health team?

The community psychiatric team includes doctors, nurses, social workers, psychologists, occupational therapists, physiotherapists and others who have different skills in assessing and enhancing the abilities of the affected person. These include: help in understanding and coping with the condition, rebuilding confidence, providing support, education about the disorder, and counselling.

What can I do to help my situation? (if the patient asks this question)

Seek professional advice from your GP and your care coordinator or psychiatrist. There are also voluntary organisations that help and advise patients suffering from schizophrenia, e.g. MIND, National Schizophrenia Fellowship and SANE, whose local contact numbers can be available from the above professional or your local Yellow Pages directory. We will get you an information leaflet on schizophrenia. It has a list of self-help groups, support groups, books and websites with information for patients as well as carers.

BIPOLAR AFFECTIVE DISORDER

Task: Mrs Smith, a 32-year-old office clerk has recently recovered from her first episode of mania and is awaiting discharge. She wants to talk to you more about the nature of the illness, the aetiology, signs and symptoms, prognosis and the treatment options. She is planning to start a family.

Suggested approach

- Greet the patient and introduce yourself.
- Explain the purpose of the visit.
- Obtain permission before you proceed.
- Build a rapport and address the patient's main concerns first.

Note: This could be asked as a complex/paired station, where in the first half of the scenario you will be asked to discuss with the patient or with the patient's relative about bipolar disorder, and in the second half of the scenario, you may have to allay patients anxiety about planning to start a family and discuss the risks involved.

Can you tell me more about my diagnosis?

You have been suffering from a manic episode. It is usually a short-lived illness, which, with treatment, you would expect to recover from in a couple of months. However, people who have had a period of mania also suffer from the other side of the illness, which is depression. Since it often occurs in the same person, the illness is called 'manic-depressive illness'. It is also called 'bipolar disorder' because there are the two poles of mania and depression.

Can you tell me more about the 'mood swings'?

We all experience minor changes in our mood from one day to the next. We may feel happy or sad. There is usually a good reason for these changes and our mood is appropriate for what is happening in our lives at the time. However, people who have bipolar disorder tend to have major changes in mood for no obvious reason. The mood changes involved in bipolar disorder range from one extreme to another. At one extreme the person may feel excessively happy and excited with a huge increase in energy and activity. This condition is called 'mania'. At the other extreme, the person may be severely depressed with a great loss of interest or energy. These mood swings usually last anywhere from a few weeks to a few months.

How common is bipolar disorder?

Bipolar disorder is quite a common illness. About one person in 100 will develop this disorder at some time in their lives. The disorder usually starts before the age of 30 but may occur at any time in the lifespan. Women and men are equally likely to be affected.

How does the doctor know I have bipolar disorder?

There is no specific medical test that can be carried out to decide whether someone has bipolar disorder. Blood tests, X-rays, or other medical tests cannot detect this disorder. This disorder can only be diagnosed by observing your behaviour and by listening to what you and your family say about your pattern of moods and behaviours.

What causes bipolar disorder?

There is no known cause but bipolar disorder is probably caused by a number of factors including heredity, chemical imbalance in the brain and stress.

Heredity

We know that this disorder can be inherited and runs in families. These findings suggest that there is likely to be some kind of faulty gene or genes in the body. If someone in the family has bipolar disorder, other family members are more likely to develop it than people who do not have a relative with bipolar disorder. However, just because one member of the family has this disorder does not mean that all family members will develop it.

Chemical disturbance

People with this disorder seem to have a chemical imbalance in the brain. It is likely that the faulty gene causes the body to produce the wrong balance of chemicals.

Stress

Stressful life events may increase the chance of developing bipolar disorder among those who are at risk. Stressful events may also make further phases of mania and depression more likely among those who already have this disorder.

What are the symptoms of mania?

In an episode of mania, you may feel:

- Very happy and excited
- Full of energy, very active

- Unable or unwilling to sleep

- Behaving in a bizarre way, recklessly spending your money, less inhibited about your social and sexual behaviour

- Speaking very quickly and jumping very quickly from one idea to another

- Full of new and exciting ideas and making plans that are grandiose and unrealistic

- Making odd decisions on the spur of the moment, sometimes with disastrous consequences.

When someone is in the middle of a manic episode, they usually do not realize that there is anything wrong with them. It is often friends, family or colleagues who first notice that there is a problem. Unfortunately, the sufferer will often object if anyone tries to point this out and when a sufferer has recovered from one of these episodes, they will often regret the things that they did and said while they were 'high'.

Will I get depressed in the future?

Bipolar disorder usually (but not always) involves episodes of depression. Although you must have had phases of mania before you can be said to have bipolar disorder; you do not need to have phases of depression to have this disorder. Most people with bipolar disorder do, however, have periods of depression at some point in their lives.

How do you know that I am depressed?

When you are depressed you may experience the following symptoms:

- Feeling sad, and miserable

- Loss of energy and greatly decreased levels of activity

- Loss of pleasure and interest in things that you used to enjoy

- Loss of appetite or weight or interest in sex

- Changes in sleeping behaviour (usually sleeping less and waking early)

- Bleak and pessimistic views of the future

- Thoughts of killing or harming yourself

- Loss of self-confidence.

For more information about the depressive phase, please see the chapter on depression.

What are mixed episodes?

This is a confusing condition for both doctors and patients to recognize. Most often, the episode is recognized as only mania or depression, only later to be recognized as 'mixed'.

Common symptoms of a mixed episode:

- Many symptoms of both mania and depression

- Very volatile mood, going from laughter to tears or anger in seconds

- Sometimes it includes mostly the physical symptoms of mania (increased energy, little need for sleep) and the emotional symptoms of depression (sadness, intense despair).

What will happen in the long run?

It is impossible to make future predictions. Each episode of mania, depression, or mixed phase lasts for a while and then stops. The person usually feels completely well again.

The length of time that a person remains well between episodes of illness varies from one person to the next. Some people may have only two or three episodes of illness and other people may have more episodes of illness. The good news, however, is that with regular medication you can reduce or even prevent further episodes of illness.

How severe is this illness?

The severity of illness differs from one person to another and even in the same person; severity varies from one episode to the next. Some episodes may be so severe that the person needs to spend time in hospital. Other episodes could be very mild and may not need hospital care and with early treatment, the episode of illness is likely to be less severe and hospital admission may be avoided.

How is this illness treated?

Bipolar disorder involves a chemical imbalance in the brain. This disturbance can be treated with medications, which are called 'mood stabilizers'. But before that, learning to cope with mood swings is vital, and many people have found that sensible life changes can also help. One of the most commonly used mood stabilizers is lithium and there are also other mood stabilizers.

Let me tell you more about lithium. Lithium is a naturally occurring substance, given as a tablet, which is an effective way of preventing mood swings for many people. It can also strengthen the effect of antidepressants. A psychiatrist usually starts treatment with lithium; although once it is stabilized it may be taken over by a GP.

How long will it take to work?

It can take 3 months or longer for lithium to work properly, so you may have to be patient and persistent in taking the tablets when nothing very much seems to be happening.

What are the side effects of lithium?

These can happen in the first few weeks after starting lithium treatment. They can be irritating and unpleasant, but often disappear or get better with time. They may include:

- Feeling thirsty
- Passing more urine than usual
- Blurred vision, dry mouth, bad metallic taste in the mouth
- Slight muscle weakness
- Occasional loose stools
- Fine trembling of the hands
- A feeling of being mildly ill
- Weight gain.

If the level of lithium in your blood is 'too high' you will experience vomiting, blurred vision, slurred speech and may feel unsteady to walk. If this happens you must contact your doctor immediately.

Do I need any blood tests?

At first you will need blood tests every few weeks to make sure that you have enough lithium in your blood, but not too much. You will need to have these tests for as long as you take lithium, but less often after the first few months. You will also need to have blood tests every few months to make sure that your kidney and thyroid gland are working properly.

Are there any dietary restrictions?

You should eat a well-balanced diet and, especially, drink regular amounts of unsweetened fluids. By doing this you can make sure you have a proper balance of salts in your body. Try to eat regularly and avoid drinking too much tea, coffee or cola. These all contain caffeine – this makes you urinate more than usual and so can upset your lithium levels.

What if I want to become pregnant?

If you become pregnant, it's usually best to stop lithium, but it is essential to ask your doctor about this. There is some evidence to show that during the first 3 months, women taking lithium may be in some danger of interfering with the baby's development. The risk appears to be low, but it is sufficient for doctors to advise the discontinuation of lithium during the early stages of pregnancy. It is therefore important to tell your doctor if you become pregnant, and it is advisable to discuss the effects of lithium and pregnancy before conception. Further, it is advisable not to breastfeed if you need to take lithium.

You may possibly suffer a relapse after childbirth. The chances are about 1 in every 3 women who have suffered from manic depression have a relapse after childbirth. I will be happy to discuss that with you, and if you wish, with your husband also.

What will happen if I stop taking the tablets?

It may be tempting to stop taking the tablets before your doctor recommends, either because of the side effects or because you don't seem to need them any more. This is unwise; bearing in mind how catastrophic the consequences can be of a manic episode. One way of feeling better about continuing with the treatment is to discuss this with your doctor and your family when you are well. You can decide in advance how you want to be treated when you are ill.

What are the chances of me getting another episode of mania or depression?

If you are thinking about the chances of having either an episode of mania or depression in the future, it is about 50/50. It is impossible to make future predictions. But in the longer run most people do have another period of depression or mania.

How can I help myself with this illness?

- **Learn to recognize the onset of mania or depression.** The switch from normal to manic behaviour often happens in a very short space of time. It is possible to learn to recognize your own early warning signs of illness. You can then seek medical help straight away – quick action can often stop the illness from becoming too severe.

- **Knowledge.** Find out as much as you can about your illness and how you can be helped.

- **Stress.** Avoid stressful situations – we know that these can trigger off a manic or depressive episode. We can't avoid all stress in our life, so it's also helpful to learn how to handle stress better. You can do relaxation training yourself with audiocassette tapes; join a relaxation group or seek advice from a clinical psychologist.

- **Relationships.** Episodes of depression or mania can cause great strain on friends and family – you may find that you have to re-build some relationships after such a time. It's important that you have at least one person that you can rely on and confide in. When you are well you should explain the illness to people who are important to you, so that they know what to expect and understand it.

- **Activities.** It is vital to balance your life between work, leisure and relationships with your family and friends. Make sure that you have enough time to relax and unwind. If you are unemployed, think about taking courses or doing some volunteer work that has nothing to do with mental illness.

So should I carry on the treatment?

You should certainly carry on the treatment for a longer period of time and it will need to be reviewed by psychiatrists in outpatients.

What should I do now?

I would recommend you to find out more about manic depression, perhaps by joining an organisation like the Manic Depression Fellowship. I will also give you some information leaflets about bipolar disorder, which you can go through when you have time, and come back to me if you have any more queries.

Note: It is worth mentioning at the end about information leaflets, fact sheets and other information available in books and on the Internet.

The issues in the Box would need to be discussed for a woman with bipolar disorder, who is already on lithium treatment and is intending to become pregnant.

Risk to the mother:

- Risk of non-compliance as she might stop her medications if she wants to get pregnant

- Risk of possible relapse during pregnancy if the treatment is stopped

- Risk of puerperal psychosis/postnatal mental illness following birth of child. The risk of relapse following delivery is significantly more, especially in the first month postpartum

- Risk of harm to self (poor self-care, self-neglect, self-harming behaviour and lack of obstetric care)

- Stress involved during pregnancy, labour and upbringing that could precipitate relapse.

Risks to the newborn

- Risks involved during pregnancy due to the effects of medication (i.e.) abortion, congenital abnormalities, teratogenic effects like Ebstein's anomaly

- Risk of harm to baby following childbirth ranging from child neglect to infanticide if mother relapses

- Risks of child inheriting the disorder from the mother (the chances of getting the illness to first-degree relatives is 10%)

- The mental health of the mother may influence fetal well being, obstetric outcome and child development (may affect the cognitive and emotional development of the infant).

DEPRESSION

Task: Mr Smith, a 30-year-old office clerk has recently recovered from his first episode of major depression and is awaiting discharge. He wants to talk to you more about the nature of the illness, the aetiology, signs and symptoms, prognosis and the treatment options.

Note: This could be asked as a 'linked/paired' station, where in the first half of the scenario you will be asked to elicit symptoms of depression, and in the second half of the scenario, you may have to discuss with the patient's relative about this condition.

Suggested approach

- Greet the patient and introduce yourself.
- Explain the purpose of the visit.
- Obtain permission before you proceed.
- Build a rapport and address the patient's main concerns first.

What is depression?

Most of us feel sad or miserable at times. These feelings may follow a disappointment, losses, or a number of other stressful or unpleasant life events. These feelings of sadness are very common and are experienced by everyone.

We recover quite quickly from our sadness, especially if we have other good things happening in our lives. Some people, however, continue to feel extremely miserable for long periods of time, even though there may no longer be a good reason for feeling this way, and may find it difficult to get through the day.

Although there is a tendency to label all our unpleasant feelings as 'depression', there are clearly some people whose depression is much more severe than others. Severe depression that occurs for no obvious reason, or that continues for a long time, at least for a period of 2 weeks is called 'major depression' or a 'depressive disorder'.

How common is depression?

Depression is a common and treatable illness. Research evidence shows that up to 25% of the population may suffer from this disorder at some time in their lives. Most cases of depression are mild, but about one person in 20 will have a moderate or severe episode. It can affect people from any age group and females are affected more commonly than males.

What are the symptoms of a depressive disorder?

1. Feeling miserable. This misery is present for much of the day but may vary in its intensity. The individual usually looks sad and 'down' and may cry often

2. Loss of interest or pleasure in usual activities, which you as a person, used to enjoy

3. Loss of appetite with excessive loss of weight

4. Loss of interest in sex

5. Loss of energy, and greatly decreased levels of activity

6. Loss of sleep despite feeling exhausted. Sleep is typically restless and unsatisfying with early morning wakening (1–2 hours earlier than usual)

7. Slowed or inefficient thinking with poor concentration, leading to difficulties sorting out problems or making plans or decisions

8. Bleak and pessimistic views of the future

9. Thoughts of killing or harming yourself

10. Loss of self-confidence

11. Slowed activity and speech.

Any of these features may serve as a warning signal of depression although many may also occur in disorders other than depression.

What causes depression?

No one knows exactly what causes depression. There is no one cause for depression and it varies greatly from one person to another. Depression seems to run in families. It seems that some people have a set of genes that makes them more likely to develop a depressive disorder.

Another factor in the cause of depression is that depression involves a chemical imbalance in the brain. Although the balance may be right most of the time, at other times the balance may change and the person becomes depressed.

Stressful life events also seem to play a part in the onset or relapse of depression. In vulnerable people these unpleasant and stressful life events may be enough to cause or worsen a depressive illness.

An individual's personality characteristics may also be an important factor. Some people have a tendency to view things in a negative way even when they are not depressed. In other words, they may have a depressive personality style. People with this kind of personality style may be at greater risk of developing a depressive disorder.

Another possible cause of depression that should not be overlooked is physical illness or medications. Certain physical illnesses, other substances of abuse, or other medications such as those for heart or blood pressure conditions, may all cause symptoms of depression.

How can I get help?

If you find that your depression is going on for more than a couple of weeks, that it is getting worse or that it is interfering with your normal activities, you should see your family doctor. Most people suffering from depression get the help they need from their GP. He or she can work out, with you, what sort of help is going to be most useful. In mild depression, counselling may be all that is needed.

What is counselling?

This is a way of talking over your problems with someone, a counsellor, who is not involved in your daily life. He or she can help by listening and allowing you to talk frankly in a way that it is sometimes difficult to do with family and friends. A counsellor may be able to help you to get a more helpful perspective on your problems. Putting feelings into words can help you to think about them more clearly, and to find practical and constructive ways of overcoming problems.

What is the treatment for moderate and severe depression?

For moderate depression medications such as antidepressants and talking treatments may be needed. For severe depression, antidepressants are usually necessary before talking treatments can be of help, and it usually needs the help of a specialist, a psychiatrist. Only a small number of people with depression ever need admission to hospital. They tend to have depressions that are life threatening or are just not getting better.

What will happen if I am left untreated?

If left untreated, depression can be so bad that life may not seem worth living. You may feel like ending the pain by **killing yourself**. If you find yourself in this situation, you must get help by telling your partner, your friend or relative, a professional, GP or the Samaritans.

What are the treatment options available?

Since depression is affected by psychological factors and may involve changes in body chemistry, depression is usually best treated by medical treatment with drugs, psychological or talking treatments and sometimes, a combination of both.

Medical treatments include antidepressant medication, electroconvulsive therapy (ECT) in severe depression, and psychological treatments including cognitive and behavioural therapy, and learning how to cope with stress.

Can you tell me briefly about antidepressants and what they are used for?

These are a number of different types of antidepressant drugs and these drugs will usually relieve depressive symptoms in most people and may help to prevent relapse of the illness. Antidepressants do not relieve your depression straight away. These drugs take some time to have an effect on your mood.

In the first few days the drugs tend to have a calming effect. However, after a week or two of taking the medication regularly, this calming effect gives way to increasing alertness and energy. It may take **6–8 weeks** before the maximum benefits of antidepressant medication are noticed. Therefore, you should not expect to notice the benefits from this medicine too quickly.

How long do I need to take these medications?

This is difficult to say but continue taking the medication for about **6 months to 1 year after recovery**. Even when you are feeling better it is important to carry on taking the tablets as your GP or psychiatrist advises. If you stop them too soon, this will make it more likely that you will become depressed again. The general rule is that you should carry on taking antidepressants at least for 6 months after your depression has lifted.

What is psychotherapy or talking treatment? Is it the same as counselling?

No, it is not the same as counselling. It is much **more structured**. There are a number of different kinds of psychotherapy or talking treatments that are useful for people who are depressed.

There are three useful forms of psychotherapy:

1. Cognitive therapy

2. Behavioural therapy

3. Interpersonal therapy.

What am I likely to gain from cognitive therapy?

People who are depressed tend to feel as if they are a **'hopeless failure'**. Cognitive therapy is a type of talking treatment that aims to help people **identify their negative ways of thinking** and teach them how to think in a more positive way. People learn that they have some control over what happens to them. They learn to bounce back from failure more effectively and to recognize and take credit for the good things in their lives.

Will they try to change the way I behave in behavioural therapy?

Depressed people lack motivation and they often sit for hours, thinking about their problems. Behavioural therapy aims to identify and change aspects of behaviour that cause or prolong symptoms of depression. Some forms of behavioural change include **activity planning, problem solving, goal planning, and social skills training.**

What is interpersonal therapy? Do you mean that I have problems with my personality?

No, not at all. This form of therapy aims to help people resolve one or more of their interpersonal problems that may be causing or prolonging symptoms of depression. For example, interpersonal therapy may target the adjustment to difficult life situations and may help with the resolution of **interpersonal disputes** (e.g. marital problems or disputes with family members at home (or) with colleagues at work).

How can I help someone who is depressed? (If the relative asks this question)

- Family and friends often want to know what they can do to help. Family members can help one another to cope with difficulties and stressful life situations.

- Being a good listener is very important. Reassurance that they will come out the other side is invaluable, though it will usually have to be repeated often as depressed people lack confidence and are prone to worry and doubt. So try to be as patient and understanding as possible.

- Spending time with depressed people, encouraging them not only to talk but to take their medications and involve them in activities, is worthwhile.

- Above all, if the depressed person is getting worse and has started to talk of not wanting to live, or even hinting at self-harm, take these statements seriously and insist that their doctor is informed. Try to help the person to accept the treatment.

Note: It is worth mentioning at the end about information leaflets, fact sheets and other information available in books and on the Internet.

POSTNATAL DEPRESSION

Task: You are seeing Ms Turner, a 30-year-old married high school teacher. Her elder sister had a baby boy 2 years ago, followed by a severe postnatal depression (PND). It improved with outpatient antidepressant drug treatment for 3–4 months. She is 2 months' pregnant now. She is worried that she might also suffer from postnatal depression as her sister did. Address the patient's concerns and allay her anxiety.

Note: This could be asked as a 'linked/paired' station, where in the first half of the scenario you will be asked to elicit symptoms of postnatal depression, and in the second half of the scenario, you may have to discuss with the patient's relative about this condition.

Suggested approach

- Greet the patient and introduce yourself.

- Explain the purpose of the visit.

- Obtain permission before you proceed.

- Build a rapport and address the patient's main concerns first.

Can you tell me about postnatal depression?

Postnatal depression (now often called PND) means becoming depressed after having a baby and it is one of the common complications following childbirth. It is like other kinds of depression except that '**it is brought on by having a baby**'.

How common is it?

It is quite common, yet often unrecognized. One out of every 10 women suffers from PND.

When does it happen?

It usually starts within 1 month of the delivery but can start up to 6 months later. It can go on for months, or even years, if untreated.

Is it not the same as baby blues?

PND is a lot different from baby blues. Many women, at least one in two would feel a bit weepy, flat and unsure of themselves on the 3rd or 4th day after having a baby. We call this 'baby blues' or 'maternity blues'.

This soon passes. Many women are weary and a bit disorganized when they get home from hospital, but they usually feel on top of the situation in a week or so. However, if it gets worse or lasts more than 2 weeks we have to consider PND.

What are the symptoms of PND?

The symptoms of postnatal depression are the same as those experienced in a depressive episode. Symptoms include:

- Depressed mood, feeling low, unhappy and tearful
- Exhaustion and loss of energy
- Sleep and appetite disturbance
- Feelings of guilt/incompetence/hopelessness
- Suicidal thoughts, plans, or actions
- Loss of libido
- Anxiety and exaggerated fears concerning the self, the baby or the partner.

The mother may feel irritable towards other children, occasionally to the baby and especially to the partner. She may feel unable to cope with the baby, unable to handle and feed the baby and may feel guilty about it. She may feel anxious and that anxiety may also make the mother concerned about her own health and worry about the baby's health.

What causes PND?

We don't know the exact cause of PND. Probably there isn't a single cause, but a number of different stresses may have the same consequence, or may act together.

We know that among these risk factors are:

1. Previous history of depression (especially PND)
2. Lack of support from the partner and family
3. Recent stressful life events
4. An accumulation of misfortunes such as bereavement, the partner losing his job, housing and money problems, etc.
5. The mother's loss of her own mother when a child.

However a woman can suffer from PND when none of these apply and there is no obvious reason at all.

Could it be hormonal?

It seems likely that huge hormone changes take place at the time of giving birth, but this evidence is still lacking. Levels of oestrogen, progesterone and other hormones to do with reproduction, which may also affect emotions, drop suddenly after the baby is born. However, women who do, and who do not, get PND have similar hormone changes.

Would mothers with PND harm the baby?

No, they don't. In fact, many mothers, even those without any mental health problems, can sometimes feel like 'throwing the screaming monster out of the window'. Mothers with PND often worry if they might harm their babies, but they never do.

However, there is another serious mental illness called puerperal psychosis, when there is a risk of the mother harming the baby. In this illness, the mother may be convinced or deluded that the baby is evil and she might harm the baby. But fortunately, this is a much rarer condition, affecting only two out of every 1000 mothers.

What treatments are available?

Since PND is similar to depression, the treatment is also similar:

- Usually, the mother may need only reassurance, practical support and supportive counselling. We can assist by organising help with childcare, placing the woman in touch with support organisations and helping the woman to recruit support from family and friends.

- We have self-help and support groups available locally. They encourage mutual support and advice regarding mothering, childcare and dealing with depression.

- If depression is associated with marital problems, they will have to be tackled through marital counselling. Give the woman permission to talk openly about her relationship with her partner and about any disappointments or stresses she may be experiencing with her new role.

- One of the most important aspects of treatment is educating new fathers. Educate the partner about postnatal depression and the demands of being a mother. Point out to the partner that the woman is in need of practical and emotional support and deal with specific relationship problems.

- It is also very important to address her social difficulties, her needs and provide adequate social support.

- For some, antidepressant drugs will be needed. In very severe cases, other drugs and even ECT may be needed.

Can I breastfeed when taking the medication?

Yes. You need not necessarily stop breastfeeding. We can find an antidepressant that does not get into your milk and affect your baby in any way.

What are the chances of me getting PND?

The chance of someone without a history of depression getting a PND is 10–15% and someone who already had one episode of PND getting a second one is higher – around 20–40%.

Are there ways to prevent it?

Yes, there are some ways to prevent it. Some of the common strategies of prevention and early intervention include:

1. Prenatal education – This education would include information about postnatal depression and this can enhance the couple's ability to recognize postnatal illness and to seek appropriate assistance if required, thereby preventing or minimising serious disability and distress.

2. Encourage the mother to keep in touch with the GP, to attend antenatal classes, take your partner with you and also to keep in touch with the health visitor.

3. Encourage the importance of regular exercise, rest, sleep, nutritious food; maintaining good relationships with your partner and family is important.

4. Techniques such as relaxation training, confidence building courses and assertiveness training may be useful for preventing the escalation of stress and help them to cope with difficult situations. Some researchers have found that psychoeducation and support programmes can halve the chances of getting a second PND.

5. Additionally, it is also recommended that women take steps to enhance their social network prior to birth if the present social network is inadequate. Advise mothers to arrange for extra support at home for at least 2 weeks, either friends, family, or professional help.

Can PND in the mother affect the baby?

Research evidence shows that PND adversely affects mothering, bonding mother–infant relationship and the emotional development of the infant. That is why we have to diagnose and treat PND as early as possible.

I will give you some information leaflets about postnatal depression, which you can go through when you have time, and I will be happy to discuss this with your husband also.

ALCOHOL – PROBLEMS, RISKS AND MOTIVATION

Task: Mr Hughes is a 43-year-old man admitted to the medical ward with gastro-oesophageal reflux disease. Counsel this patient about the risks of excessive alcohol intake and ways to deal with this problem.

Note: This could be asked as a 'linked/paired' station, where in the first half of the scenario you will be asked to elicit symptoms of alcohol history, and look for features of alcohol dependence and in the second half of the scenario, you may have to discuss with the patient about the harmful effects of alcohol misuse.

Suggested approach

- Greet the patient and introduce yourself.
- Explain the purpose of the visit.
- Obtain permission before you proceed.
- Address his main concerns.
- Start with open questions.
- **Do not take an alcohol history.**

Alcohol is our favourite drug. Most of us use it for enjoyment, but for some, drinking can become a serious problem.

Let us discuss 'sensible drinking'?

It is a good idea for all of us to keep track of how much we drink. We can do this by counting the number of units we drink in a week. A unit is the amount of alcohol found in half a pint of beer, lager or cider; a short of whisky or other spirits; and a small glass of wine or sherry.

If you drink less than 21 units a week for a man or 14 for a woman, you probably will not have a problem – as long as you spread it out across the week. You should also give yourself at least two alcohol-free days each week. It is wise not to drink more than 2 units in any one day for a woman and more than 3 units in any one day for a man.

We all tend to underestimate the amount we drink. One way of finding out exactly how much we are drinking is to keep a diary for a week, writing down each day how much we have had to drink. If we do this every now and then we can check how much alcohol we are actually drinking by adding up our score in units.

Drinking too much alcohol can cause physical health problems, mental health problems and social problems.

How can it affect our physical health?

Alcohol irritates the stomach walls and can cause gastritis. It can make stomach ulcers worse. Drinking too much over a long period of time can cause liver disease and increases the risk of some kinds of cancer in the liver.

Being very drunk can lead to severe hangovers, and can cause tears on the food pipe resulting in massive bleeding, vomiting blood, unconsciousness and even death.

How can it affect the liver?

The liver has to work hard to get the alcohol out of the body. After a certain period the liver becomes exhausted and it starts failing. This can cause hepatitis and jaundice. After some time it starts shrinking, causing **cirrhosis** of the liver, which kills the person.

What else can it do to our body?

Alcohol can affect each and every system in the body. It can damage the pancreas and interfere with blood glucose. Alcohol can affect the muscles of the heart and can even cause **heart** problems. It can affect your mental health as well.

Can alcohol affect our mental health?

Excess drinking itself is a mental heath problem. Alcohol is a very common cause of depression, anxiety and sleep problems. Many people who take overdoses and kill themselves have an alcohol problem and they do so whilst drunk.

In fact, alcohol causes all sorts of sexual problems including loss of erection. In some people alcohol can cause them to hear imaginary voices. This is usually a very unpleasant experience and can be hard to get rid of. Alcohol can stop your memory from working properly and in extreme cases cause brain damage.

In what ways can it affect the brain?

Alcohol is toxic to the brain cells. When people drink too much for too long, the nerve cells are affected and they can die off. This can cause memory loss and dementia.

Alcohol also affects the nerves outside the brain, for example in the legs and arms. This affects the sensations in our body, which we call peripheral neuropathy.

What else can it do to people?

Alcohol is the commonest cause for people ending up in casualty with falls, accidents, broken bones or head injury. Excessive drinking can cause accidents at home, on the roads, in the water and on playing fields.

Many problems are caused by people having too much to drink at the wrong place or time. They include: fights, arguments, money troubles, family upsets, and spur-of-the-moment casual sex.

Alcohol is a very common reason for domestic violence and family break-ups. Often alcohol becomes the most expensive thing in people's lives. Many people get into serious debt because of their drinking.

Alcohol can make you do things you would not normally do. Sometimes people get into trouble and are convicted for drunken driving or drunk and disorderly behaviour.

What are the warning signs of excessive drinking?

Alcohol is addictive. It is a bad sign if you find you are able to hold a lot of drink without getting drunk. You know you are hooked if you do not feel right without a drink, or need a drink to start the day.

How can I change the habit of excessive drinking?

I am really pleased that you have asked this question. We all find it hard to change a habit, particularly one that plays such a large part in our lives. There are three steps to dealing with the problem:

1. Realising and accepting that there is a problem.

2. Getting help to break the habit.

3. Keeping going once you have begun to make changes.

We can help you to deal with alcohol problems.

What sort of help is available to deal with alcohol problems?

- Initially it may be enough to keep a diary of your drinking and then to cut down if you find you have been drinking too much.

- It helps if you can talk your plans over with a friend or relative. Do not be ashamed to do that. Most real friends will be pleased to help and you may find they have been worried about you for some time.

Getting help

- If you find it hard to change your drinking habits then try talking to your GP or go for advice to a counsel on alcohol.

- Your GP can refer you to the Local Drug and Alcohol Team.

- If you still find it very difficult to change then you may need specialist help.

- Groups where you meet other people with similar problems can often be very helpful. Groups may be self-help types like Alcoholics Anonymous, or arranged by an alcohol treatment unit.

- For some people, a short time in an alcohol treatment unit might be helpful.

Are there any drugs available to treat this problem?

If you feel you cannot stop because you get too shaky or restless and jumpy, then your doctor can often help with some medication for a short time.

Drugs are not used very often at first except for 'drying out' (also known as 'detoxification'). It is important to avoid relying on tranquillizers as an alternative.

Although beating a drink problem may be hard at first, most people manage it in the end and are able to lead a normal life.

- It is worth mentioning about information leaflets and fact sheets at the end of the consultation.

ALZHEIMER'S DISEASE

Task: Mr Spencer White is the son of an 82-year-old (Mr White) who was recently seen in the 'memory clinic'. Mr White lives with his 80-year-old wife. He was referred to the clinic by his GP, and following assessment and further investigations the diagnosis of early Alzheimer's disease was made. Mr Spencer White has made an appointment to see you to discuss his father's condition. Explain the nature, aetiology, signs and symptoms, treatments and likely outcomes of his father's condition.

Note: This could be asked as a 'linked/paired' station, where in the first half of the scenario you will be asked to elicit collateral history of dementia, and in the second half of the scenario, you may have to discuss with the patient's relative about this condition.

Suggested approach

- Greet the patient and introduce yourself.
- Explain the purpose of the visit.
- Obtain permission before you proceed.
- Build a rapport and address the relative's main concerns first.

Thank you for seeing me, doctor. Can you tell me exactly what is wrong with my father please?

As you know your family doctor has had concerns about your father's memory. We saw him in the memory clinic. After our assessment, we found that he has definite memory difficulties and we carried out some tests and the results obtained suggest that his memory problems are most likely to be due to a type of dementia called 'Alzheimer's disease'.

What is dementia?

Dementia is the name given to a group of diseases that affect the normal working functions of the brain. Although the causes are largely unknown, the effects are all too familiar: a progressive, irreversible destruction of brain cells that leads to memory loss, confusion, personality and behaviour changes. Alzheimer's disease is one among them.

What is Alzheimer's disease?

Alzheimer's disease is the commonest type of the dementias. Everyone loses brain cells, as they get older. In people with Alzheimer's disease, this process is more severe and rapid than in normal ageing. The parts of the brain that deal with memory are usually affected first. The onset of this illness tends to be gradual.

Loss of short-term memory is usually the first noticeable sign. Patients become increasingly forgetful and slowly other parts of the brain are affected. In the later stages people may develop problems with their speech or undertaking practical tasks.

How common is this condition?

It affects 5% of people over the age of 65. Both males and females are affected. Although it mostly affects people over 65, it can also occur in young people. With younger sufferers, there is often a family history. But in most instances it is not inherited.

What tests have you done to confirm that he has Alzheimer's disease?

Making a definite diagnosis of Alzheimer's disease while the person is still alive is difficult. Only at postmortem can a diagnosis be confirmed. So a thorough medical and psychiatric assessment is always essential.

- 'We interviewed your parents to obtain a clear history of his problems and we also assessed his mental state.'

- 'We did a thorough physical and neurological examination, which did not reveal any signs of physical illness.'

- 'We did some blood tests to exclude conditions that can sometimes cause memory loss; these were all normal.'

- 'We referred him to the clinical psychologist, who assessed his memory and other brain functions in detail. These tests also showed that your father does have clear problems with memory.'

- 'Finally, we did a CT brain scan, which showed some changes in his brain tissue.'

What will happen in the early stage?

In the early stages a person with dementia often appears confused and forgetful about things that have just happened. He or she may not remember what they did 5 minutes ago, or where they are. Long-term memory tends to stay intact and for this reason people with dementia often dwell in the past. Also, in the early stages, concentration and decision making become difficult.

Mood changes are also frequent. A previously happy person may become irritable or depressed over little things. As the disease progresses, confusion, forgetfulness and mood changes become much more obvious. Those affected may become anxious and aggressive, and may wander aimlessly around the house.

Personal safety is also very much at risk, especially for those who smoke or cook. Even simple things like dressing become difficult. The stress upon carers is enormous, as it becomes difficult to leave someone alone for even a few minutes.

What will happen in the final stages?

In the final stages of the disease, people with dementia need a great deal of help. Often they are unable to **recognize** even close family and friends. Communication is frequently a problem: the ability to talk clearly and understand what is being said is often lost. Incontinence is common, and those affected often become bedridden or wheelchair-bound. Because of this, many sufferers finally die from an infection or virus such as pneumonia.

Does that mean he is definitely going to get worse?

Unfortunately, it is a progressive condition. The illness cannot be halted or reversed; ultimately I'm afraid that he will deteriorate.

How long has he got to live?

Most studies have shown people to live for 5–10 years after being diagnosed. However these are only rough and average figures and it really is impossible to make firm predictions in individual patients. What we can assure you at this moment is your father's illness is relatively mild at present and he is in good physical health for his age.

What sort of help can you offer with looking after him?

We can offer him help in various different ways:

- First of all, we will be seeing your father in the 'memory clinic' to monitor his response to the drug treatment.
- We have also arranged for one of our community nurses to visit your parents at their home. Both you and your mother will be able to contact her for advice. If your father needs any urgent medical input, she will contact us and make arrangements for it.
- She will work with our social worker to ensure that your parents receive all the benefits to which they are entitled, and that they are offered appropriate practical help.

What is a memory clinic and what are they likely to do?

Memory clinics are specialist outpatient clinics set up specifically to diagnose and often treat people complaining of memory problems. They have the ability to investigate, diagnose and treat people suffering from memory problems with antidementia drugs and also monitor their response to treatment periodically.

What sort of help can social services offer?

- If your father needs help with personal care, such as washing or dressing, then a Home carer can visit to assist him.

- Social services can arrange for him to attend a day centre to provide him with some company and to allow your mother to have a break.

- Often outside help in the form of meals on wheels, home help etc. make it possible for people to maintain some independence, dignity and privacy.

- The local occupational therapists should be able to supply bath equipment, banister rails, a wheelchair, and special seating (if necessary in the future) and these can be obtained through social services.

- Sitting services can sometimes be provided to enable the carer to have a short break from caring.

- The social services are able to provide short stays of 1–2 weeks in a residential home to provide relatives a short period of respite.

- Respite care over a longer period can also be provided to give the carer a break from their caring role, maybe for a holiday.

- If a stage comes where your mother cannot manage to care for your father at home then social services can help to organize permanent care in a suitable residential or nursing home.

What is a community care assessment?

The carer who looks after the patient with Alzheimer's disease may be entitled to help from social services, including things such as personal care, adaptations or equipments for the home. The first important step in making sure that the patients get the help from statutory services is having their 'needs assessed', which is also called community care assessment.

Following the assessment, the carer will be told about what services are available and a **care package** can then be set up with their agreement and that of the person they care for.

What about financial and legal arrangements?

As dementia progresses, people become increasingly unable to manage their own affairs. Informal arrangements often exist to get around this problem: a friend or relative collects benefits and pensions. It is important, however, to get legal advice before any major problems arise.

In the early stages of the disease the person with dementia may be competent enough to appoint somebody with Power of Attorney for managing his or her affairs. A solicitor can arrange this. However, if the person's mental capacity is too limited for a valid Power of Attorney, it may be necessary to put his or her affairs under the jurisdiction of the Court of Protection.

The following are able to offer help on legal and financial issues: Citizens' Advice Bureau, Mind, Alzheimer's Disease Society's legal advisor, or any solicitor.

Can he drive?

This is a very common problem faced by the patients who suffer from dementia and will become more so as people who are regular car users get older.

Not everyone with dementia is banned from driving but if a person has a severe degree of cognitive impairment it is dangerous for him or her to do so and it is strictly not advisable as the rights of the individual to drive are outweighed by the risk to others.

If your father has been given a diagnosis of dementia, he must inform the DVLA about it or you or any member of the family can do this on his behalf. The final decision will be taken by the DVLA after taking advice from the GP and specialists involved in your father's care.

Where can I obtain more information about Alzheimer's disease?

The Alzheimer's Disease Society is extremely helpful. They produce various books and leaflets. Your father can join a local self-help group to meet other people in the same position who can provide an invaluable source of practical information. Above all as his main carer, your mother will need help and support and we have invited your mother to join the relatives' support group.

Counselling/Explanation About a Particular Drug or Treatment

ELECTROCONVULSIVE THERAPY TO THE PATIENT

Task: You are seeing Mr Jones, a 55-year-old man suffering from a major depressive disorder. He has been treated with two different antidepressants on adequate dosage and for adequate duration (6 weeks) but has not improved. He did comply with these treatments. Your consultant has proposed that he is treated with ECT.

You are asked to give the patient information about ECT with a view of assisting him to decide whether or not he is willing to agree to have ECT. You are not required to assess his capacity to give consent.

Note: This could be asked as a 'linked/paired' station, where in the first half of the scenario you will be asked to explain ECT treatment and obtain consent, and in the second half of the scenario, you may have to administer ECT treatment to a mannequin.

Suggested approach

- Greet the patient and introduce yourself.

- Explain the purpose of the visit.

- Obtain permission before you proceed.

- Build a rapport and address the patient's main concerns first.

What does ECT stand for?

ECT stands for 'electroconvulsive therapy'.

Why is ECT used?

Most people who have ECT are suffering from depression. Although we have a variety of different tablets for depression some people do not recover completely and others take a long time. ECT is often used for these patients. In severe cases of depression, ECT may be the best treatment and it can be life saving.

Why has ECT been recommended for me?

ECT is given for many reasons. It may be very helpful if you did not get better with antidepressant drugs. The other situations where it is very helpful are:

- ECT is most commonly used to treat severe depression not responding to drug treatment.

- It may be helpful if you can't take antidepressant drugs because of the side effects.

- It may help if you have responded well to ECT in the past.

- It may help if you feel so overwhelmed by your depression that it's difficult to function at all, and that your life is in danger because you are not eating (or) drinking enough and wishing to kill yourself.

Is it not a barbaric treatment?

No, not at all. Owing to the advances in the field of anaesthesia and with modern equipment, ECT has become more sophisticated and you may not experience any pain or suffering. People show good improvement following ECT treatment.

What will actually happen when I have ECT?

The treatment takes place in a separate room and only takes a few minutes. The anaesthetist will ask you to hold out your hands so you can be given an anaesthetic injection. It will make you go to sleep and cause your muscles to relax completely. You will be given some oxygen to breathe as you go off to sleep. Once you are fast asleep, a small amount of electric current is passed across your head and this causes a mild fit/seizure in the brain. There are little movements of your body because of the relaxant injection that the anaesthetist gives. When you wake up, you will be back in the waiting area and there will be a nurse accompanying you.

What will happen immediately before the treatment?

An ECT treatment involves having an anaesthetic. You will need to fast (have nothing to eat and drink) from about midnight the night before each treatment. This will involve having no breakfast or tea or coffee on the morning that you have ECT.

How will I feel immediately after ECT?

Some people wake up with no side effects at all and simply feel very relaxed. Others may feel somewhat confused or have a headache. There will be a nurse with you when you wake up after the treatments to offer you reassurance and make you feel as comfortable as possible.

How does ECT work?

The exact mechanism is not known.

During ECT, a small amount of electric current is passed across your brain. This current produces a fit/seizure, which affects the entire brain including centres that control thinking, mood, appetite and sleep. Repeated treatments alter the chemical imbalance in the brain and bring them back to normal. This helps you begin to recover from your illness.

How well does ECT work?

More than 8 out of 10 depressed patients who receive ECT respond well, making ECT the most effective treatment for severe depression. People who have responded to ECT report themselves to be more optimistic, making them feel like themselves again, less suicidal, and that life is worth living. Most patients recover their ability to work and lead a productive life after their depression has been treated with a course of ECT.

What is a course of ECT?

A course of ECT involves 6–8 treatment sessions on an average. ECT is usually given twice a week. It is not possible to say exactly how many treatments you may need. Some people get better with a few treatment sessions but others may need as many as 12 and very occasionally even more.

What are the side effects of ECT?

Some patients may be confused and get headaches just after they awaken from the treatment, and this generally clears up within an hour or so. Sometimes your memory of recent events may be upset and at times simple things may be temporarily forgotten. In most cases this memory loss goes away within a few days or weeks, although sometimes patients continue to experience memory problems for several months. But ECT does not have any long-term effects on your memory or your intelligence.

Are there any serious risks from the treatments?

ECT is amongst the safest medical treatments given under general anaesthesia; the risk of death or serious injury with ECT is rare and occurs in about one in 50,000 treatments. This is much lower than that reported for childbirth. Very rarely deaths do occur and these are usually because of heart problems. Even when you have heart problems, it may still be possible for you to have ECT safely with special precautions such as heart monitoring. We will ask another specialist to advise if there are grounds for concern.

What other treatments could I have?

Antidepressant drugs may be available to treat your particular condition and it is possible that some of them may work as well as ECT. Psychological or talking treatments are available, but they are more useful for milder forms of depression.

Will I have to give my consent? Can I withdraw my consent to have ECT?

At some stage before the treatments, we will ask you to sign a consent form for ECT. If you sign the form it means that you are agreeing to have up to a certain number of treatments (usually six). You can refuse to have ECT and you may withdraw your consent at any time, even before the first treatment has been given. The consent form is not a legal document and does not commit you to have the treatment. It is a record that an explanation has been given to you and that you understand to your satisfaction what is going to happen to you. Withdrawal of your consent to ECT will not in any way alter your right to continue treatment with the best alternative methods available.

Are there any risks in not having ECT as recommended?

If you choose not to accept your doctor's recommendation to have ECT, you may experience a longer and more severe period of illness and disability than might otherwise have been the case.

What about counselling?

This is generally more useful in milder depressions. Currently, your depression is too severe for you to benefit from them. It is not a good idea to go for counselling at this stage.

What about another drug?

ECT usually works more quickly than medication. But with regard to medication, we could try yet another antidepressant drug. However, you may have to wait for up to 6–8 weeks to know whether the new drug is effective, and there is the possibility of new side effects. Drug therapy also has risks and complications and drug treatment are not necessarily safer than ECT.

My friend had ECT in the past. She suffered memory problems and confusion. Can anything be done to reduce it?

We calculate the lowest, efficient dose for each individual patient and give treatment only twice a week, reducing this to once a week if necessary. If there are serious concerns about memory problems, instead of giving the electrical stimulus bilaterally across both temples, we can give it unilaterally to just one side of the head.

What can't ECT do?

The effects of ECT will only relieve the symptoms of depression, but will not help all your other problems. An episode of depression may produce problems with relationships or problems at home or work. These problems may still be present after your treatment and you may need further help with these. Hopefully, because the symptoms of your depression are better, you will be able to deal with these problems more effectively.

It is worth mentioning at the end about information leaflets, fact sheets and other information available in books and on the Internet.

TREATMENT WITH ATYPICAL ANTIPSYCHOTICS

Task: Mr Williams is a 30-year-old man admitted to the psychiatric ward with a diagnosis of paranoid schizophrenia. He is sensitive to conventional anti-psychotics and develops extrapyramidal side effects. Your consultant has decided to start him on an atypical antipsychotic, preferably olanzapine. Explain to the patient about the drug and address his concerns.

Suggested approach

- Greet the patient and introduce yourself.

- Explain the purpose of the visit.

- Obtain permission before you proceed.

- Build a rapport and address the patient's main concerns first.

Note: The following questions and answers can be used for any of the atypical antipsychotics except the side effect profile, which is clearly explained at the end of this section.

What are atypical antipsychotics used for?

These drugs are generally used to help treat illnesses or conditions, such as psychosis and schizophrenia. These drugs seem to be equally effective at the proper dose, but have fewer side effects than the older drugs.

How do they work?

There is a naturally occurring chemical in the brain called 'dopamine'. Dopamine is the chemical messenger mainly involved with thinking, emotions, behaviour, and perception. In some people, dopamine may be overactive and upset the normal balance of chemicals. Excess dopamine helps to produce some of the symptoms of the illness. The main effect of these drugs is to block some dopamine receptors in the brain, reducing the effect of having too much dopamine, and correcting the imbalance. This reduces the symptoms caused by having too much dopamine.

When should I take them?

Take your medication as directed by the doctor. Try to take them at regular times each day. Taking them at mealtimes may make it easier for you to remember, as there is no problem about taking any of these drugs with or after food. If the instructions say to take them once a day, this is usually better at bedtime, as they may make you drowsy at first, but they are not sleeping tablets.

How long will they take to work?

Some of the effects of these drugs appear soon after taking them, for example, the drowsiness. The most important action, to help the symptoms of your illness, may take days to weeks of regular medication to become fully effective. Similarly, if your dose or treatment is changed, it may take an equally long period of time before you notice the effects of such a change.

For how long will I need to keep taking them?

This is quite difficult to say at this moment, as people's responses are different. You will probably need to continue your treatment for a long time, possibly even for several years after your symptoms have disappeared, to make sure you have fully recovered from your illness. Long-term treatment should be reviewed at regular intervals, for example, every 3–6 months or even sooner if there are problems.

Are they addictive?

These drugs are not really addictive. If you have taken them for a long time, you may experience some mild effects if you stop taking them suddenly. The main problem would be your symptoms returning.

Can I stop taking them suddenly?

It is unwise to stop taking them suddenly, even if you feel better. Your symptoms can return if treatment is stopped too early. This may occur some weeks or even many months after the drug has been stopped. When the time comes, we will usually withdraw the drug by a gradual reduction in the dose taken over a period of several weeks.

What sort of side effects might occur?

Like other drugs, these drugs may cause adverse effects. Some are relatively mild and occur during the initial adjustment period. These can happen in the first few weeks after starting the treatment. They can be unpleasant but often disappear or get better with time. Some of the common side effects are:

Side effect	What happens
Drowsiness	Feeling sleepy or sluggish
Dry mouth	Not much saliva or spit
Constipation	You cannot pass a motion
Hypotension	Low blood pressure – this can make you feel dizzy
Weight gain	Eating more and putting on weight

The good thing is that these newer medications do not have the unpleasant side effects of restlessness, muscle stiffness, and shakes but they are equally effective.

Will they make me drowsy?

These drugs may make you feel drowsy or sleepy. You should not drive (see below) or operate machinery until you know how they affect you. You should take extra care, as they may affect your reaction times or reflexes. However, they are not sleeping tablets, although if you take them at night they may help you to sleep.

Will they cause weight gain?

Weight gain with these drugs is quite possible and more likely with olanzapine. In the people who gain weight, most is gained during the first 6–12 months of treatment. It then tends to level out. It is not possible to say what the effect on your own weight may be because each person will be affected differently. If you do start to put on weight or have other problems, you should tell your doctor. He/she may be able to adjust your drug or the dose of your drug to reduce this effect. Your doctor can also arrange for you to see a dietician for advice. If you do gain weight, it is possible to lose it while you are still taking this medication, with expert advice about diet.

Will it affect my sex life?

Drugs can affect desire (libido), arousal (erection), and orgasmic ability. These drugs are not thought to have a significant effect on any of these stages, but problems have been reported occasionally with these drugs. If this happens, however, you should discuss it with your doctor, as a change in dose or drug may help to minimize the problem.

Can I drink alcohol while I am taking these drugs?

If you drink alcohol while taking these drugs it may make you feel sleepier. This is particularly important if you need to drive or operate machinery, and you must seek advice on this.

Are there any foods or drinks that I should avoid?

You should have no problems with any food or drink other than alcohol.

Will they affect my other medication?

You should have no problems if you take other medications, although a few problems can occur. Sedative drugs might make you feel sleepier. This does not necessarily mean the drugs cannot be used together, just that you may need to follow your doctor's instructions very carefully. You should tell your doctor before starting or stopping these, or any other drugs. Make sure your doctor knows about all the medicines you are taking.

What should I do if I forget to take them?

Start again as soon as you remember, unless it is nearly time for your next dose, and then take the next dose as normal. Do not try to catch up by taking two or more doses at once, as you may experience more side effects. If you have problems remembering your doses (as many people do) ask your pharmacist, doctor, or nurse about this. There are some special packs, boxes, and devices available that can be used to help you remember.

If I were to take a contraceptive pill, will this be affected? (female patients)

It is not thought that 'the pill' is affected by any of these drugs.

Will I need a blood test?

Not usually.

Can I drive when I am on this drug?

These drugs can affect your driving, e.g. you may feel drowsy. Until this wears off or you know how your drug affects you, do not drive or operate machinery. You should take extra care, as they may affect your reaction times or reflexes, even though you feel well.

It is an offence to drive, attempt to drive, or to be in charge of a vehicle when unfit through drugs. It is advisable to let your insurance company know if you are taking these drugs. If you do not and you have an accident, it could affect your insurance cover.

Note: It is worth mentioning at the end about information leaflets, fact sheets and other information available in books and on the Internet.

- Ask whether the patient has any more questions.

- Thank the patient and the examiner.

Common side effects of antipsychotic medications

Here are the names of antipsychotic medications used commonly in clinical practice and their side effects:

Typical or older antipsychotics (e.g. chlorpromazine, haliperidol, etc.) – sedation, hypotension, autonomic side effects like dry mouth, constipation, blurred vision, urinary retention, impaired ejaculation, extrapyramidal side effects (EPSEs) like akathisia, tremors, weight gain and ECG changes.

Atypical or newer antipsychotics

Olanzapine – drowsiness, dry mouth, constipation, hypotension, oedema, weight gain, impaired glucose tolerance

Risperidone – insomnia, agitation, anxiety, headache, nausea, abdominal pain, weight gain, sometimes EPSEs, increased prolactin levels causing amenorrhoea, galactorrhoea, loss of libido, breast engorgement

Quetiapine – dizziness, drowsiness, postural hypotension, dry mouth, weight gain

Amisulpride – insomnia, agitation, nausea, constipation, increased prolactin levels causing amenorrhoea, galactorrhoea, and loss of libido, breast engorgement, osteoporosis

Clozapine – dizziness, drowsiness, constipation, weight gain, hypersalivation, tachycardia, fever, neutropenia/agranulocytosis, seizures

Aripiprazole – Constipation, akathisia, headache, nausea, vomiting, stomach upset, agitation, anxiety, insomnia, sleepiness, lightheadedness, tremor

Zotepine – Dry mouth, constipation, dyspepsia, tachycardia, headache, agitation, anxiety, QT interval prolongation, weight gain, sexual dysfunction.

CLOZAPINE TREATMENT

Task: Mr Taylor is a 44-year-old man with a diagnosis of chronic schizophrenia resistant to treatment, and he has been on various combinations of medications without much benefit. Your consultant has suggested that he should be started on clozapine. Explain how you would commence him on clozapine and discuss the potential benefits and side effects of clozapine.

Suggested approach

- Greet the patient and introduce yourself.
- Explain the purpose of the visit.
- Obtain permission before you proceed.
- Build a rapport and address the patient's main concerns first.

For what is clozapine used?

Clozapine is one of the newer antipsychotic drugs used to treat symptoms of schizophrenia in people who have not done well on at least two other similar drugs, e.g. who have not responded or who have had unpleasant side effects.

How does clozapine work?

There are many naturally occurring chemical messengers ('neurotransmitters') in the brain and dopamine is one of them. Dopamine is the chemical messenger mainly involved with thinking, emotions, and behaviour. In schizophrenia, it may be overactive, which helps to produce some of the symptoms of the illness. The main effect that clozapine has is to block some of the dopamine in the brain, reducing the effect of having high levels, and reducing the symptoms caused by too much dopamine.

Will I need a blood test?

Clozapine can upset the blood of about two or three in every 100 people taking it. It can reduce the number of white cells or neutrophils in the blood. This makes it much harder for your body to fight infections. You must, therefore, have regular blood tests for as long as you are taking this medicine.

How often are these blood tests done?

You will need a test before you start clozapine, then every week for the first 18 weeks, and every 2 weeks from then on. If you have been taking clozapine regularly for 1 year without any blood problems, it may be possible to change the blood tests to every 4 weeks. The blood is usually posted to the Clozapine Patient Monitoring Service, which returns the results to the pharmacy and doctor.

You may also need extra blood tests if it is thought that your blood is being affected. You must not miss these tests. Your doctor and pharmacist will not be able to let you have any more tablets if you do.

Remember the rule: no blood, no tablets.

When should I take clozapine?

Take your clozapine as directed by your doctor. Try to take it at regular times each day. Taking it at mealtimes may make it easier to remember, as there is no problem in taking clozapine with or after food. If the instructions say to take it once a day, this should usually be at bedtime, as it may make you feel drowsy when first taking it, although clozapine is not a sleeping tablet.

How long will clozapine take to work?

Some effects of clozapine, such as drowsiness, appear soon after taking it. The most important action, helping to control the symptoms of your illness, may take several weeks to months, or even up to 1 year, of regular medication to become fully effective. In the same way, if your dose or treatment is changed, it may take an equally long time before you notice the effects of such a change.

For how long will I need to keep taking it?

This is very difficult to tell, as people's responses are different. However, you will probably need to continue your treatment for several years. Long-term treatment should be reviewed every 3–6 months or sooner if there are problems. It is likely that you will benefit from clozapine by taking it for many years.

Is clozapine addictive?

Clozapine is not addictive. There is no evidence whatsoever to indicate that people taking clozapine become physically dependent on the medication.

Can I stop taking clozapine suddenly?

It is unwise to stop taking clozapine suddenly, even if you feel better. Your symptoms can return if treatment is stopped too early. This may occur some weeks or even many months after the drug has been stopped and we call it 'rebound psychosis'.

What should I do if I forget to take it?

Start again as soon as you remember unless it is almost time for your next dose, then goes on as before. Do not try to catch up by taking two or more doses at once, as you may experience more side effects. If you have problems remembering your doses (as many people do) tell your pharmacist, doctor, or nurse about this. There are special packs, boxes, and devices available that can be used to help you remember.

What sort of side effects might occur?

Like other drugs, clozapine may cause adverse effects. Some are relatively mild and occur during the initial adjustment period. These can happen in the first few weeks after starting the treatment. They can be unpleasant, but often disappear or get better with time. Some people taking clozapine may experience no adverse effects at all.

Some of the common side effects are:

Common side effect	What happens
Drowsiness	Feeling sleepy or sluggish
Constipation	Difficulty in passing a motion
Hypersalivation	Your mouth is full of saliva and you may drool
Hypotension	Low blood pressure – this can make you feel dizzy
Weight gain	Eating more and putting on weight
Fever	Rise in body temperature
Palpitations	A rapid heart beat

Are there any dangerous side effects?

One of the more serious side effects is that it can reduce the number of white cells or neutrophils in the blood, resulting in a condition called 'neutropenia'. This makes it much harder for your body to fight infections. On higher dosage, it can also induce a seizure or a fit.

Warning signs

If you think you have a cold, sore throat or any other infection, tell your doctor or nurse immediately. They will arrange a blood test to check your white cell count. If your white cell count is normal you should be able to continue with your treatment, but your doctor will tell you if this is the case.

Will clozapine make me drowsy?

Clozapine may make you feel drowsy or sleepy. You should not drive or operate machinery until you know how it affects you. You should take extra care, as it may affect your reaction times or reflexes. Clozapine is not, however, a sleeping tablet, although if you take it at night it may help you to sleep.

Will clozapine cause weight gain?

When you start taking clozapine, you may experience weight gain. This tends to stop after a time, but can be a problem with clozapine. It is thought that the drug causes an increase in appetite, which then makes you eat more and put on weight. If you do start to put on weight, or have problems with your weight, you should tell your doctor. The doctor may be able to change your clozapine dose to reduce this effect. Your doctor can also arrange for you to see a dietician for advice. Any weight you put on can be controlled while you are still taking this drug, with expert advice about diet. Make sure your doctor knows about this if it causes you distress.

Will clozapine affect my sex life?

Drugs can affect desire (libido), arousal (erection), and orgasmic ability. Unlike many other antipsychotic drugs, clozapine has not been reported as having a major adverse effect on the three stages, except by causing drowsiness. However, if this happens, you should discuss it with your doctor, who may recommend a change in dose to help minimise the problem.

Can I drink alcohol while I am taking clozapine?

You should avoid alcohol while taking clozapine, as it may make you feel sleepier. This is particularly important if you need to drive or operate machinery. You must seek advice on this.

Are there any foods or drinks that I should avoid?

You should have no problems with any food or drink other than alcohol.

Will it affect my other medication?

You should have no problems if you take other medications, although some have been recorded. Clozapine should not be taken with some antibiotics, e.g. co-trimoxazole and chloramphenicol. It can also interact with a few other drugs, including some drugs for depression and some anticonvulsants, e.g. carbamazepine. This does not necessarily mean the drugs cannot be used together, just that you may need to follow your doctor's instructions very carefully. Make sure your doctor knows about all the medicines you are taking. You should tell your doctor before starting or stopping these or any other drugs.

If I am taking a contraceptive pill, will this be affected? (Female patients)

It is not thought that the contraceptive pill is affected by clozapine. With many drugs of this type, a woman's periods may be irregular or even disappear. This is less likely with clozapine and so they may reappear or become more regular if changing to clozapine.

Can I drive while I am taking clozapine?

Clozapine can affect your driving in two ways. Firstly, you may feel drowsy and/or suffer from blurred vision when starting to take the drug. Secondly, clozapine can slow down your reactions or reflexes. This is especially true if you also have a dry mouth, blurred vision, or constipation (the so-called 'anticholinergic' side effects). Until these effects wear off, or you know how your clozapine affects you, do not drive or operate machinery. It is advisable to let your insurance company know if you are taking clozapine. If you do not and you have an accident, it could affect your insurance cover.

Who organizes the blood monitoring?

The Clozapine Patient Monitoring Service organizes the monitoring. Its main aim is to make sure patients being treated with clozapine are regularly monitored to reduce the risk of any adverse effects on their white cell levels. This way they can alert your doctor quickly if there is a problem. This service keeps track of the progress of every single patient taking clozapine and keeps up-to-the-minute records of all blood test results.

What form does monitoring take?

Before clozapine is started, a blood test is carried out to check that your white cell count is satisfactory. Then, if all is well, your doctor will start treatment. When treatment starts you will be monitored.

Regular blood testing is the main form of monitoring. You will have a blood test every week for at least 18 weeks. After 18 weeks all your blood results will be reviewed, and if all is well, testing may change to every second week until the end of the first year of treatment.

The risk of neutropenia decreases after the first year of treatment. If your blood tests have been satisfactory, you should be able to transfer to testing every 4 weeks. Testing will then continue every 4 weeks for as long as you are taking clozapine.

What happens if you miss a blood test?

Because of the risk of neutropenia, there is one very important rule about taking clozapine tablets – no blood result, no drug treatment.

How will you start my treatment?

When we want to start anyone on clozapine treatment we have to register the patient. Once you are registered, treatment can begin.

As with other antipsychotic medicines, clozapine can cause some general side effects. To keep these unwanted effects to a minimum, we will start you on a low dose and increase it slowly as well as adjusting the dose depending on how you react. This way of tailoring medicines to an individual is called titration. The aim of titrating clozapine in this way is to achieve the best effect with the minimum of unwanted side effects at the lowest effective dose.

Normally, we will start you on 12.5 mg once or twice on the first day. On the second day you will have one or two 25 mg tablets. If necessary, the daily dose can be increased further by 50–100 mg, usually in half-weekly or weekly intervals, up to a maximum of 900 mg per day.

How long will it take before the medicine begins to work and does it work for everyone?

Some people feel the benefit of their treatment within a few days while other people can wait from a few months to a year. Therefore, it's important to be patient and give your treatment a chance to work.

About six out of 10 people will benefit from taking clozapine. Some do very well and others will be a bit better. Unfortunately, some people do not respond to the medicine, but they will not be made any worse by trying it.

How will I know the medicine is working?

You may notice that you feel better and are becoming less withdrawn and able to be more involved in life around you.

You will probably find that your relatives, friends or carer notice the reduction in your symptoms before you.

How long the medicine should be taken for?

Clozapine should continue to be taken every day as prescribed for as long as you are benefiting from taking it. Treatment should not be stopped because your symptoms have diminished or disappeared. If you stop taking clozapine the symptoms are quite likely to come back.

Just like any prescribed medicine your doctors must see you regularly. If your doctor feels you should stop taking clozapine, for reasons other than neutropenia, withdrawal from the drug should be done slowly over a period of time.

What happens if I miss one dose?

If you miss a dose take your next dose at the normal time. Do not try to make up the missed dose by taking more. Do not double dose.

What happens if I miss more than one dose?

If you have missed more than 48 hours of your medicine, you must contact your nurse or doctor immediately. You must not carry on with the same dose as before. It is essential to start again from 12.5 mg once or twice on the first day under the supervision of your doctor. However, if you tolerated the initial doses of clozapine well, your doctor may be able to increase the dose to your maintenance level more quickly.

Pregnancy and breastfeeding (women)

The safety of clozapine during pregnancy is not clear and therefore should not be taken. Clozapine is also thought to get through to breast milk and so mothers taking clozapine should not breastfeed their babies.

Note: It is worth mentioning at the end about information leaflets, fact sheets and other information available in books and on the Internet.

- Ask whether the patient has any more questions.

- Thank the patient and the examiner.

ANTIDEPRESSANT TREATMENT (SELECTIVE SEROTONIN RE-UPTAKE INHIBITORS)

Task: You have seen Mr Hughes in the outpatients' clinic and he has been diagnosed as suffering from depression. You are planning to start him on paroxetine (SSRI). Explain to the patient about the drug and address his concerns.

Suggested approach

- Greet the patient and introduce yourself.
- Explain the purpose of the visit.
- Obtain permission before you proceed.
- Build a rapport and address the patient's main concerns first.

Note: The following questions and answers can be used for any of the SSRIs.

What are SSRIs?

SSRIs are selective serotonin re-uptake inhibitors.

What is paroxetine?

Paroxetine is one of the SSRIs, which belong to a class of antidepressants.

What are SSRIs used for?

SSRIs are antidepressants that are used to help improve mood in people who are feeling low or depressed. All these drugs are sometimes used to help other illnesses, e.g. anxiety, bulimia nervosa, panic attacks, and obsessive–compulsive disorder.

SSRIs are now one of the most commonly prescribed antidepressants, but there are many other similar drugs. All these antidepressants seem to be equally effective at the proper dose, but have different side effects from each other. SSRIs generally have fewer side effects than the older drugs. If one drug does not suit you, it may be possible to try another.

How do SSRIs work?

The brain has many naturally occurring chemical messengers. One of these is called serotonin and this is important in the areas of the brain that control mood and thinking. It is known that serotonin is not as effective or active as normal when someone is feeling depressed. SSRI antidepressants increase the amount of the serotonin chemical messenger and this can help to correct the lack of action of serotonin and improve mood.

When should I take them?

Take your medication as directed by your doctor. If you are told to take your dose once a day this will usually be better in the morning. If you feel sick when first taking the SSRI, this should only last for a few days, but taking the medication with or after food can relieve the nausea. Also, taking the SSRI at **mealtimes** may be easier to remember, and there are no problems about taking any of these drugs with or after food. However, they are not sleeping tablets.

How long will they take to work?

It may take 2 weeks or more before the SSRIs start to have any effect on your mood, and a further 3–4 weeks for this effect to reach its maximum. If it has not started working in about 6 weeks, it is less likely to work. Unfortunately, in some people, the effect may take even longer, e.g. several months, especially if you are older.

For how long will I need to keep taking these tablets?

This is very difficult to say, as people's responses are different. To help you make a decision, it may be useful for you to know that research has shown that:

- For a first episode of major depression, your chances of becoming depressed again are much lower if you keep taking the antidepressant for 6 months after you have recovered (longer if you have risk factors for becoming depressed again).

- For a second episode, your chances of becoming depressed again are lower if you keep taking the antidepressant for 1 or 2 years after you have recovered.

- For depression that keeps returning, continuing to take an antidepressant has been shown to have a protective effect for at least 5 years.

When the time comes, your doctor should withdraw the drug slowly, e.g. by reducing the dose gradually every few weeks.

Are SSRIs addictive?

SSRIs are not addictive, but if you have taken them for 8 weeks or longer, you may experience some mild 'discontinuation' effects if you stop taking them suddenly. These do not mean that the antidepressant is addictive but these are more of an 'adjustment' reaction from sudden removal of the drug rather than withdrawal.

Can I stop taking them suddenly?

It is unwise to stop taking it suddenly, even if you feel better. Two things could happen. Firstly, your depression can return if treatment is stopped too early. Secondly, you may experience some mild 'discontinuation' symptoms.

What are 'discontinuation' symptoms?

These could include: dizziness, vertigo/light-headedness, nausea, fatigue, headache, 'electric shocks in the head', insomnia, agitation, and anxiety. These can start shortly after stopping or reducing doses, are usually short-lived, will go if the antidepressant is started again, and can even occur with missed doses. These effects have been reported for all the SSRIs, but seem to occur more often with paroxetine than the others.

What should I do if I forget to take a dose?

Start again as soon as you remember, unless it is almost time for your next dose. Do not try to catch up by taking two or more doses at once, as you may experience more side effects.

If you have problems remembering your doses (as many people do) ask your pharmacist, doctor, or nurse about this. There are special packs, boxes, and devices available that can be used to help you remember.

What sort of side effects might occur?

Like other drugs, these drugs may cause adverse effects. Some are relatively mild and occur during the initial adjustment period. These can happen in the first few weeks after starting the treatment. They can be unpleasant but often disappear or get better with time. Some of the common side effects are:

Common side effect	What happens
Nausea and vomiting	Feeling sick and being sick
Insomnia	Not being able to fall asleep at night
Restlessness or anxiety	Feeling tense and nervous, and possibly sweating more
Headache	A pounding and painful head
Loss of appetite	Not feeling hungry, and possibly losing weight
Diarrhoea	Passing loose, watery stools
Sexual dysfunction	Finding it hard to have an orgasm. No desire for sex

Will the drugs make me drowsy?

These drugs may make you feel drowsy, although this effect is less compared with other antidepressants. You should not drive or operate machinery until you know how they affect you. You should take extra care, as they may affect your reaction times or reflexes.

Will the drugs cause me to put on weight?

The other drugs in this group tend to have less effect on body weight. However, if you do start to have problems with your weight tell your doctor at your next appointment, who can then arrange for you to see a dietician for advice.

Will the drugs affect my sex life?

Drugs can affect desire (libido), arousal (erection), and orgasmic ability. The SSRIs are known to affect **all three stages** in some people. Delayed orgasm is known to occur in many people. Indeed some of these drugs are now widely used to help treat premature ejaculation. If this does seem to be happening, you should discuss it with your doctor, as a change in drug dose or the time when you take the dose may help to reduce problems.

Can I drink alcohol while I am taking the SSRI?

You should avoid alcohol except in moderation while taking these drugs as they may make you feel sleepier. This is particularly important if you need to drive or operate machinery, and you must seek advice on this.

Are there any foods or drinks that I should avoid?

You should have no problems with any food or drink other than alcohol.

Will the SSRI affect my other medication?

You should have no problems if you take other medications, although a few can occur. The SSRIs can 'interact' with other antidepressants and blood thinners, e.g. warfarin. This does not necessarily mean that the drugs cannot be used together, but you may need to follow your doctor's instructions very carefully. Make sure your doctor knows about all the medicines you are taking. You should tell your doctor before starting or stopping these, or any other drugs.

If I am taking a contraceptive pill, will this be affected?

It is not thought that the contraceptive pill is affected by any of these drugs.

Will I need a blood test?

You will not need a blood test to check on your SSRI.

Can I drive while I am taking the SSRI?

You may feel drowsy at first when taking any of these drugs. Until this wears off, or you know how the drug affects you, do not drive or operate machinery. You should take extra care, as they may affect your reaction times.

It is an offence to drive, attempt to drive, or to be in charge of a vehicle when unfit through drugs. It is advisable to let your insurance company know if you are taking these drugs. If you do not and you have an accident, it could affect your insurance cover.

Note: It is worth mentioning at the end about information leaflets, fact sheets and other information available in books and on the Internet.

- Ask whether the patient has any more questions.

- Thank the patient and the examiner.

Common side effects of medications

Here are the names of common antidepressant medications used commonly in clinical practice and their possible side effects.

Selective serotonin reuptake inhibitors

Fluoxetine, paroxetine, citalopram, escitalopram, sertraline.

a. Gastrointestinal side effects
Nausea, vomiting, dyspepsia, abdominal pain, diarrhea.

b. Central nervous system side effects
Headache, sweating, anxiety, agitation, insomnia, sexual dysfunction.

c. Sexual side effects
Loss of libido, erectile dysfunction.

Newer antidepressants

Venlafaxine
Nausea, headache, dry mouth, insomnia, dizziness, sweating, somnolence, sexual dysfunction, elevation of blood pressure at higher doses.

Duloxetine
Nausea, dryness of mouth, constipation, diarrhoea, vomiting, decreased appetite, dizziness, somnolence, insomnia.

Mirtazapine

Headache, nausea, dizziness, increased appetite, weight gain, drowsiness, oedema.

Reboxetine

Insomnia, sweating, dizziness, dry mouth, constipation, tachycardia, urinary hesitancy.

Older antidepressants

Tricyclic antidepressants (e.g. amitryptyline, imipramine, clomipramine, dothiepin)

Sedation, hypotension, autonomic side effects like dry mouth, constipation, blurred vision, urinary retention, impaired ejaculation, weight gain, ECG changes and arrhythmias.

Trazadone and nefazodone

Nausea, drowsiness, dizziness, postural hypotension, fatigue, headaches, anticholinergic side effects such as dry mouth, constipation and elevation of hepatic enzymes.

Irreversible monoamine oxidase inhibitors (MAOIs) (isocarboxazid, phenelzine, tranylcypromine)

Drowsiness, insomnia, agitation, dizziness, weakness, fatigue, diarrhea, weight gain, edema, postural hypotension and anticholinergic side effects.

Reversible inhibitor of monoamine oxidase type A (RIMA) – moclobemide

Nausea, headache, dizziness, insomnia, anxiety, restlessness, dry mouth, blurred vision, rash.

LITHIUM CARBONATE

Task: Mr Green is a 30-year-old man who has just recovered from a manic illness, treated under section. He had a similar manic episode 10 years ago and a depressive episode 4 years ago. Your consultant has suggested he take lithium prophylaxis. Explain to the patient the rationale of taking lithium and the practicalities of lithium therapy.

Suggested approach

- Greet the patient and introduce yourself.

- Explain the purpose of the visit.

- Obtain permission before you proceed.

- Build a rapport and address the patient's main concerns first.

When is lithium used?

Lithium is a mood stabilizer. Lithium is used in treating and controlling mood disorders like depression and mania, especially when they keep coming back. It is also used to increase the effect of antidepressant drugs when these are not working enough on their own.

Lithium tends to lead to fewer manic and depressive episodes or to their disappearance. Even if these still occur the mood swings are usually less severe, but it may take several months or even years to control mood swing.

What is lithium?

Lithium is a substance that occurs naturally in food and water. Small amounts can therefore be found in the body. However, this does not mean that it is a natural substance everybody needs, and it is therefore important to note that lithium is not given because people have a deficiency of the substance. Certain minerals have high lithium content and it is from this source that the medication lithium salts are made.

Are there any precautions to be taken prior to beginning lithium treatment?

Yes. Before beginning lithium therapy, your doctor will need some information that includes your medical history including heart disease, thyroid disease, kidney disease, psoriasis or epilepsy or any history of mental health problems in your family, especially mania or depression.

Also tell your doctor about any medications you are taking, especially diuretic medications (water pills used to treat high blood pressure), drugs used for asthma, painkillers, steroids and antidepressants.

Are there any tests to be done prior to commencement of lithium therapy?

It may be necessary for you to undergo a number of tests to ensure that the medication can be used safely, and these include:

- **Kidney function test:** An evaluation of how your kidneys function is essential because lithium is eliminated from your body in the urine.

- **Thyroid function test:** A test of the thyroid function is also important because lithium may interfere with the thyroid function and may cause under activity or over activity of the thyroid gland. Once on lithium, a thyroid test is recommended every 6 months.

- **Heart function test:** People who have a history of severe heart disease should not be given lithium. Therefore we also do ECG, which is the tracing of the heart to find out if there are any major heart problems before starting the patient on lithium treatment.

- **Blood tests:** Once you have begun treatment, it will also be necessary to have regular blood tests (sometimes called 'a lithium level', a 'serum lithium level' or a 'plasma lithium level'). This test is important because it enables the doctor to monitor the amount of lithium in the bloodstream, and therefore ensures that your dosage is both effective and safe.

Doses are adjusted to keep the blood level within the range of 0.4 and 1.0 mmol/L, which is considered to be the appropriate therapeutic range to maximize benefits and minimize side effects.

How long do we need to have blood tests?

Blood tests are needed more often in the early stages of treatment or when your dosage is adjusted. In these circumstances, they may be needed at least once a week. Once serum levels have stabilized, they will be needed only once a month and even less frequently later. As a rough guide, blood tests should be done at least every 3 months once serum levels have stabilized.

Are there any dietary restrictions to be followed while on lithium?

Making sure that the body is provided with proper amounts of salt and water is a very important part of lithium therapy. Here are a few guidelines:

- **To maintain water balance:** drink at least four to six pints of fluid each day. Avoid excessive amounts of coffee, tea or cola drinks containing caffeine. Caffeine causes water loss and can interfere with lithium therapy.

- **To maintain salt balance:** ensure that your diet contains an average amount of salt. Inform your doctor before you begin any new diets, especially low salt diets. Do not fast while taking lithium.

- **To avoid excessive loss of both water and salt:** take special care to avoid situations where you are likely to sweat heavily, such as too much activity in hot weather, exposure to sauna baths, and heavy exercise.

What are the side effects of lithium therapy?

Like other drugs, lithium may cause adverse effects. Some are relatively mild and occur during the initial adjustment period. These can happen in the first few weeks after starting lithium treatment. They can be irritating and unpleasant, but often disappear or get better with time. Many people taking lithium experience no adverse effects at all.

Some of the early adverse effects may include:

- Feeling thirsty
- Passing more urine than usual
- Blurred vision
- Dry mouth
- Bad metallic taste in the mouth
- Slight muscle weakness
- Occasional loose stools
- Fine trembling of the hands
- A feeling of being mildly ill.

Are there are any long-term side effects?

Some of the long-term side effects are:

1. Excessive weight gain
2. Changes in kidney functioning, which may lead to damage
3. Thyroid changes: Reduced thyroid activity can cause sleepiness, tiredness, lethargy, slowed thinking, feeling cold, headache, dry skin, constipation, muscle aches, unusual weight gain or conversely increased thyroid activity or hyperactivity
4. Shaky hands
5. Skin rash.

However, these side effects can be prevented and controlled by regular blood tests, and monitoring.

Are there any dangerous side effects?

If the level of lithium in your blood is too high, you will experience:

- Persistent diarrhoea

- Severe nausea/vomiting

- Severe hand tremors

- Blurred vision

- Slurred speech

- Lack of co-ordination

- Confusion

- Frequent muscle twitching.

This means the lithium is reaching unacceptable levels within the body, and you need immediate attention to avoid serious poisoning. You have to contact your doctor immediately for advice.

Let your doctor know if you have a high fever, involving excessive sweating or vomiting or diarrhoea. It may be necessary to stop taking lithium temporarily until your physical health has returned to normal.

If I don't feel better after a few days, does this mean the medication isn't working?

No. Lithium does not always work quickly. It can take anything from a few days to several weeks for any noticeable improvement to take place. Although some people feel better as soon as they begin taking lithium, most improve more gradually.

If I am pregnant, can lithium prove harmful?

Yes, at certain stages of the pregnancy. There is some evidence to show that during the first 3 months of pregnancy, women taking lithium may be in some danger of interfering with the baby's development. The risk appears to be low, but it is sufficient for doctors to advise the discontinuation of lithium during the early stages of pregnancy. It is therefore important to tell your doctor if you become pregnant, and it is advisable to discuss the effects of lithium and pregnancy before conception.

Prospective parents should note that there are no known harmful effects on children whose fathers were taking lithium at the time of conception or earlier; or on children of women who had taken lithium before but not during pregnancy.

Is it dangerous to drink while taking lithium?

In most cases, it is safe to drink alcohol in moderation. It is best, however, to check with your doctor when starting treatment.

Does lithium interact with 'over-the-counter drugs'?

'Over-the-counter medicine' refers to medicines that are available for purchase from community pharmacies without the presentation of a medical prescription. The sale does however have to be supervised by a registered pharmacist.

Yes, it does interact with certain drugs like ibuprofen, which on higher doses have been shown to raise serum lithium levels. If you are taking or intend to take the combination of these drugs, it is very important to consult your doctor or pharmacist first. It is always a good idea to let the pharmacist know about any other medicines that you are taking, so that they can tell you of any potential problem with drug combinations.

Is lithium addictive?

No. There is no evidence whatsoever to indicate that people taking lithium become physically dependent on the medication. However, some research suggests that some people may experience a recurrence of their original symptoms when they stop taking lithium suddenly. But it is important to remember that people need support to withdraw lithium at their own pace.

Is it safe to drive while taking lithium?

This will vary from person to person. Lithium can impair co-ordination and it is therefore important to take particular care when driving or operating dangerous machinery, and stop if it is clear that you cannot do so safely.

Is it safe to exercise regularly?

It is perfectly safe to exercise regularly provided that you ensure you take in sufficient fluids and salt. It is also advisable to time your lithium dose so it is not taken immediately before vigorous exercise.

How long will it prove necessary to take lithium?

This will vary from person to person. Depending on the course of your condition lithium may prove necessary to prevent episodes of mania or depression for the rest of your life. It is not a cure for manic depression, but a preventive medication.

You should have regular reviews of your lithium treatment to discuss with your doctor whether it is still needed. Psychiatric research shows that a large proportion of lithium users will relapse if lithium is stopped, but it is not possible to tell in advance who will have further severe mood swings and who will not.

If you have been completely free of relapses for three to four years, some doctors may be willing to reduce and stop your lithium for a trial period, under close supervision.

Are there people who should avoid taking lithium?

Yes. People who have a history of kidney disease or a severe heart disease are not advised to take lithium.

Does lithium always work?

No. Some people do not respond to lithium therapy and others cannot tolerate it. Some may respond only partially, and may experience reduced or less severe episodes of depression and mania. It is important therefore that you do not raise your expectations too highly, when commencing treatment. It may take 6 months to a year to achieve a full effect as a preventive treatment.

Are there other treatments for manic depression?

If someone is particularly susceptible to lithium's unwanted effects, then there are other mood stabilizers such as carbamazepine and semisodium valproate, which can be given as an alternative, and these are sometimes given in combination with lithium if the mood swings are only partially controlled.

Some practical tips when taking lithium

- Do ensure that your diet includes plenty of salt and water. A reduction in either may allow lithium to build up to dangerous levels.

- Do inform your doctor immediately about any adverse effects you notice. Minor adverse effects can be discussed at routine sessions with your doctor, but any adverse effects mentioned previously should be reported immediately.

- Do ensure that you tell any other doctor who is treating you that you are taking lithium, or any other medication. If you are admitted to hospital for any reason, you should also tell the doctor treating you that you are taking lithium. If you are given a lithium treatment card, always remember to take this with you.

- Don't double up a dose of lithium if you forget a prescribed dose. If you have missed your regular time by 3 hours or less, take your normal dose. If you have missed your normal dose by more than 3 hours, skip the forgotten dose and resume your lithium medication at the next scheduled time.

- Don't change your prescribed dosage without consulting your doctor. The appropriate dosage will vary from patient to patient and your doctor will be in the best position to judge how much you should take.

- It is worth mentioning at the end about information leaflets, fact sheets and other information available in books and on the Internet.

- Ask whether the patient has any more questions.

- Thank the patient and the examiner.

Mood stabilizers – common side effects

Lithium

Increased thirst, polyuria, polydipsia, nausea, vomiting, abdominal pain, muscular weaknesses, tremors, weight gain, acne, hypothyroidism

Carbamazepine

Drowsiness, ataxia, diplopia, nausea, hepatitis, rashes, blood dyscrasias

Sodium valproate

Headache, nausea, vomiting, sedation, hair loss, weight gain, ataxia, and blood dyscrasias.

VALPROATE SEMISODIUM

Task: Mr Black is a 32-year-old man who is an inpatient in your ward and suffers a manic episode. He has a lengthy history of bipolar affective disorder with recurrent episodes in the past. He has been tried on other mood stabilizers without much benefit. Your consultant has decided to start him on valproate semisodium (Depakote). Explain the drug to the patient and address his main concerns.

Suggested approach

- Greet the patient and introduce yourself.

- Explain the purpose of the visit.

- Obtain permission before you proceed.

- Build a rapport and address the patient's main concerns first.

For what is valproate used?

Valproate is generally used in the treatment of epilepsy to help control fits or seizures. Valproate can also be used to help mood disorders (especially if the person is high – as an antimanic) and some other illnesses, particularly when other treatments have not been effective.

How does valproate work?

It is not entirely clear how valproate works (either as a mood stabilizer or as an anticonvulsant), as it causes several actions in the brain. There is a chemical messenger (or 'neurotransmitter') called **GABA**, which calms the brain down. In some people, it is thought that there may not be enough GABA in the brain. This lack seems to 'trigger' fits or overactivity/mania.

Valproate helps to stop the breakdown of GABA and so leaves enough in the brain thereby controlling overactivity/mania and acts as a mood stabilizer.

How long will valproate take to work?

Valproate should begin to work soon after you start taking it. It may, however, take time before your doctor finds the dose that is right for you. The aim is to achieve a level of medicine in your blood that is high enough to control overactivity, but low enough to cause the least amount of side effects. If you are taking it to help prevent mood swings, it may take weeks to months to reach maximum effect.

145

Will I need blood tests?

For the first 6 months of treatment you will need a regular blood test to check that the drug is not affecting your **liver**.

You may then need to have blood tests from time to time to ensure that the dose of valproate is enough and not too much or too little to control the condition for which it has been prescribed.

For how long will I need to keep taking valproate?

This is very difficult to say as people's responses are different. What I can say is valproate is a 'preventative medicine' and you may need to take it for a long time, several months or even years.

What will happen if I stop taking it suddenly?

Never stop taking this medication suddenly or without advice from your doctor, as this may cause an increase in your fits or your symptoms may worsen. When the time comes to stop your valproate, this is usually by a **slight reduction in your dose** every few weeks.

What sort of side effects might occur?

Like other drugs, it may cause side effects. Some are relatively mild and occur during the initial adjustment period. These can happen in the first few weeks after starting the treatment. They can be unpleasant but often disappear or get better with time. Some people may experience no adverse effects at all.

Some of the common side effects are drowsiness, feeling sick, increased appetite, weight gain, you may have an upset stomach and you may feel tired all the time. Some people also complain of hair loss, disturbed menstrual periods in women and on higher doses some patients feel unsteady on their feet.

Will valproate make me drowsy?

You may feel sleepy when you first start taking this drug, so you must take extra care if you are allowed to drive or when operating any type of machinery. This effect should wear off after you have been taking it for a while.

Will valproate cause weight gain?

Valproate can make some people feel hungry and they may put on weight. A few people may put on weight without eating more. If you start to experience weight gain or have other weight-related problems, your doctor can arrange for you to see a dietician for advice.

Will valproate affect my sex life?

Drugs can affect desire (libido), arousal (erection), and orgasmic ability. Valproate has not been reported to have a major adverse effect on these three stages. However, if this does seem to happen, you should discuss it with your doctor, as a change in dose may help minimize any problem.

Can I drink alcohol while I take valproate?

There is no complete ban on drinking alcohol if you are taking valproate, but make sure you do not have more than one or two drinks a day, as it may make you feel sleepier. This is particularly important if you are allowed to drive or operate machinery, and you must seek advice on this.

Are there any foods or drinks that I should avoid?

You should have no problems with any food or drink apart from alcohol.

Can I drive while taking valproate?

If you are allowed to drive, remember that valproate can make you drowsy when you first start taking it, so extra care should be taken when driving or operating any type of machinery. It is advisable to let your insurance company know if you are taking this drug. If you do not and you have an accident, it could affect your insurance cover.

- Ask whether the patient has any more questions.

- It is worth mentioning at the end about information leaflets, fact sheets and other information available in books and on the Internet.

- Thank the patient and the examiner.

ANTIDEMENTIA DRUGS – EXPLAIN TO A CARER

Task: Mr Bateman, a 78-year-old man, is diagnosed as suffering from mild Alzheimer's disease. The consultant has decided to start him on donepezil (Aricept). His daughter, who is also his main carer, has heard that there are new drug treatments available. She has fixed an appointment to see you to discuss more about these drugs.

Suggested approach

- Greet the patient and introduce yourself.
- Explain the purpose of the visit.
- Obtain permission before you proceed.
- Build a rapport and address the relative's main concerns first.

New drugs for dementia

I have heard that there are new drug treatments available for Alzheimer's disease. Could you tell me more about them please?

Yes. You are right. Recently some new drugs have been made available for the treatment of Alzheimer's disease. These drugs are collectively called 'antidementia drugs'. There are no major differences between these drugs. Some of the examples include donepezil (Aricept), rivastigmine and galantamine. More drugs are on the way.

How will Aricept help my father?

It will not cure him completely, but it may help to stabilize the illness or improve his condition for a while. It may help his memory. He can also have general benefits including improving alertness and motivation. More often carers see general improvements in behaviour or mood.

How effective are these drugs?

Research studies have shown that 50–60% of people who have taken these drugs have shown some improvement or stabilisation of their condition over a period of 6 months.

How do they work?

In Alzheimer's disease, one of the chemicals in the brain called 'acetylcholine', which is important for learning and memory, is in short supply.

So if you have less acetylcholine activity, then you may have less memory ability and reduced learning. The drugs act by increasing the brain levels of acetylcholine and help to stabilize or improve memory, learning and functioning.

How do you go about starting the drug?

First of all, the specialist will see him in the 'memory clinic'. People are often given a screening memory test called the 'mini mental state examination,' also called an MMSE. The total score is 30, and we suggest starting these drugs when the MMSE score lies between 10 and 20. But before that, we have to find out if the drug suits him. We will take a history, including a detailed medical history to rule out severe heart, kidney or liver problems or breathing problems and do relevant investigations necessary to rule out any treatable causes for his memory problems. Then we will also do a formal assessment of his daily living skills and if all goes well then we may start him on these drugs (like in your father's case).

How is the treatment given?

We will start with one tablet of 5 mg of donepezil (Aricept) once a day. We will need to re-evaluate this dose in about 4 weeks. We shall ask a nurse to see your father after about 2 weeks of treatment to make sure that he is not having side effects.

How long do these drugs take to work?

These drugs take at least 4 weeks to show their full effect at the starting dose. After 4 weeks, we may increase his dose.

How long would he stay on this drug for?

Initially we usually prescribe these drugs for a trial period of 3 months to see, if at the end of 3 months, your father has shown any benefits from this drug. If not we may take him off the drug.

If he does show improvement, then we will need to review him approximately every 6 months to see if it is worthwhile continuing the treatment.

The MMSE is repeated once every 6 months and we suggest stopping these drugs when the MMSE score goes below 10 out of 30. However, in some patients, if we stop the drug they may deteriorate rapidly and we may have to consider reintroducing it.

What sort of side effects may occur?

All medicines have side effects, yet some patients may experience none of them. The most common problem is feeling nauseous or a bit sick in the beginning. But it tends to disappear gradually as the body gets used to the treatment and generally will not last more than a few days. Other common side effects are loss of appetite, tiredness, muscle cramps and sometimes poor sleep.

The uncommon and rare side effects are urinary retention and seizures.

Will these drugs make him feel drowsy?

Drowsiness is not a main side effect of these drugs but if you do feel drowsy, then you should not drive or operate dangerous machinery. You should take extra care as they may affect your reaction times.

Will these drugs cause weight gain?

Weight gain is not a reported side effect of these drugs. But if it happens, tell your doctor at your next appointment.

Can he drink alcohol while he is taking these drugs?

The combination of donepezil and alcohol may cause drowsiness. However, patients on donepezil can have an occasional drink, if they wish.

Are there any dietary restrictions?

You should have no problems with your food or drink.

Will these drugs affect his other medication?

You should have no problems if you take other medications.

Will he need a blood test?

You should not need to have a blood test to check on your drug, although your doctor may want to check your blood for other reasons.

Are these drugs addictive?

These drugs are not addictive. There is no evidence of withdrawal symptoms.

I have heard the treatment is expensive. Will we have to pay for this treatment?

No, these drugs are now available on the NHS.

- Ask whether the patient has any more questions.
- It is worth mentioning at the end about information leaflets, fact sheets and other information available in books and on the Internet.
- Thank the patient and the examiner.

Antidementia drugs and side effects

Donepezil, rivastigmine and galantamine – Common side effects would include nausea, vomiting, dizziness, insomnia, and diarrhea.

Summary of NICE guidance on acetylcholinesterase inhibitors

- Acetylcholinesterase inhibitors may be prescribed for those with Alzheimer's disease with an MMSE score between 10 and 20.

- Diagnosis must be made in a specialist clinic.

- Assessments of cognitive functioning and activities of daily living should be made before starting drug treatment.

- Only specialists should initiate treatment.

- Only those likely to comply with drug treatment should be considered.

- Those remaining on drug treatment should thereafter be assessed at 6-monthly intervals. If MMSE scores indicated no deterioration or improvement and there is evidence of global or functional improvement then treatment should continue.

- Acetylcholinesterase inhibitors should not normally be used in patients where MMSE scores fall below 10 points.

DEPOT MEDICATION

Task: Mr Hill is a 46-year-old man who suffers from chronic schizophrenia. He has had multiple admissions in the past with recurrence of symptoms due to non-compliance with oral medications. Your consultant has proposed to start him on Flupenthixol depot injections (Depixol). Explain to the patient about the drug and address his concerns.

Allay the patient's anxiety first, as some patients are apprehensive of injections.

Note: The following questions and answers can be used for any of the depot medications, with some changes to the side effect profile of individual drugs.

What are depot medications?

Depots are injections, and they are a slow release form of antipsychotic. A 'depot' injection is a long-acting injection, usually given into a buttock or sometimes the thigh. If you are in hospital, a nurse will give the injection.

What are the advantages of having these injections as opposed to tablets?

The injection releases the drug slowly over several weeks, so you will not have to remember to take tablets at regular times each day. Depot injections are neither more nor less effective than tablets or capsules.

You only have to have the injection once a week or once a fortnight, or even once a month. As you will have an appointment to go to your doctor or nurse to have the injection, you can remember easily when you have to have the injection.

If you missed your injection, your doctor or nurse would remind you. Above all, it may help you with your unpleasant experiences such as hearing voices, and you may be symptom-free when you are having the injection.

Who will give the injection and where will I have my injection?

You can usually decide yourself where to have the injections. The possible choices are:

1. At your local doctor's surgery

2. At a community mental health centre

3. At a special outpatient clinic

4. At your home, when a nurse visits you.

What happens when the nurse gives the depot medication?

You will go into a private, comfortable room. Usually there will be no one except yourself and a nurse. Initially you will be given a small amount of the medicine called a 'test dose' to see if it has any bad effects on you, and to make sure the drug suits you. Then, if there are no problems, 5–10 days later you will be given your first full-dose injection, which will then be repeated every 1–4 weeks. These injections are usually given into the buttock, although some may be given into the thigh.

How do they work?

To put it briefly, these are made up of chemicals that help to balance out the chemicals in the brain. There is a naturally occurring chemical in the brain called 'dopamine'. Dopamine is the chemical messenger mainly involved with thinking, emotions, behaviour, and perception. In some illnesses, dopamine may be overactive and upset the normal balance of chemicals. Excess dopamine helps to produce some of the symptoms of the illness. The main effect of these drugs is to block some dopamine receptors in the brain, reducing the effect of having too much dopamine, and correcting the imbalance. This reduces the symptoms caused by having too much dopamine.

How do they help?

Drugs help to alleviate the most disturbing symptoms of the illness. Medication works in two ways:

1. It reduces the symptoms of an attack of the illness.

2. Once the symptoms have improved it helps prevent further attacks or the symptoms getting worse.

Why do I need a test dose?

Depots are long acting. Any adverse effects that result from injection are likely to be long-lived. Thus a small test dose is essential to help avoid severe, prolonged adverse effects.

If the medicine is OK for you, then you will start having regular injections. After each injection, the medicine will stay in your body for a few weeks.

Are there any side effects?

Like any other medication, these injections can also give you some difficulties. You may get some pain when the needle enters your skin. Other side effects are:

Common side effect	What happens
Drowsiness	Feeling sleepy or sluggish
Hypotension	Low blood pressure, feeling dizzy
Constipation	You may have some difficulty in passing motion or stools
Dry mouth	Not enough saliva or spit
Blurred vision	Things look fuzzy and you cannot focus properly
Weight gain	Eating more and putting on weight
Restlessness	Being on edge. You may feel restless
Movement disorders	Having shaky hands and feeling shaky

What should I do if I get any of these side effects?

Tell your doctor, your nurse or your key worker. They will want to help you with any problem with your medicine.

Can anything help with these side effects?

Yes. Often, having smaller amounts of the injection may help. Sometimes giving other tablets to counteract the side effects can also help.

How often do I have to have these injections?

We will administer at the longest possible licensed interval roughly between once a week and once a month.

How long will they take to work?

Some of the effects of these drugs appear soon after taking them, for example, the drowsiness. The most important action, to help the symptoms of your illness, may take weeks, or even months of regular medication to become fully effective. Similarly, if your dose or treatment is changed, it may take an equally long period of time before you notice the effects of such a change.

For how long will I need to keep taking them?

It is very difficult to say, as people's responses are different. You will probably need to continue your treatment for a long time, possibly several years after your symptoms have disappeared, to make sure you have fully recovered from your illness. Long-term treatment should be reviewed at regular intervals, for example, every 3–6 months, or even sooner if there are problems.

Are they addictive?

These drugs are not really addictive. If you have taken them for a long time, you may experience some mild effects if you stop taking them suddenly. The main problem would be your symptoms returning.

Can I stop taking them suddenly?

It is unwise to stop taking them suddenly, even if you feel better. Your symptoms can return if treatment is stopped too early. When the time comes, we will usually withdraw the drug by a gradual reduction in the dose taken over a period of several weeks.

Will they make me drowsy?

These drugs may make you feel drowsy or sleepy. You should not drive or operate machinery until you know how they affect you. You should take extra care, as they may affect your reaction times or reflexes. However, they are not sleeping tablets, although if you take them at night they may help you to sleep.

Will they cause weight gain?

Weight gain with these drugs is quite possible. In the people who gain weight, most is gained during the first 6–12 months of treatment. It then tends to level out. It is not possible to say what the effect on your own weight may be because each person will be affected differently. If you do start to put on weight or have other problems, you should tell your doctor. He/she may be able to adjust your drug or the dose of your drug to reduce this effect. Your doctor can also arrange for you to see a dietician for advice. If you do gain weight, it is possible to lose it while you are still taking this medication, with expert advice about diet.

Will it affect my sex life?

Drugs can affect desire (libido), arousal (erection), and orgasmic ability. These drugs are not thought to have a significant effect on any of these stages, but problems have been reported occasionally with these drugs. If this happens, however, you should discuss it with your doctor, as a change in dose or drug may help to minimize the problem.

Can I drink alcohol while I am taking these drugs?

If you drink alcohol while taking these drugs it may make you feel sleepier. This is particularly important if you need to drive or operate machinery, and you must seek advice on this.

Are there any foods or drinks that I should avoid?

You should have no problems with any food or drink other than alcohol.

Will they affect my other medication?

You should have no problems if you take other medications, although a few problems can occur. Sedative drugs might make you feel sleepier. This does not necessarily mean the drugs cannot be used together, just that you may need to follow your doctor's instructions very carefully. You should tell your doctor before starting or stopping these, or any other drugs. Make sure your doctor knows about all the medicines you are taking.

If I am taking a contraceptive pill, will this be affected?

It is not thought that 'the pill' is affected by any of these drugs.

Will I need a blood test?

Not usually.

Can I drive while I take them?

These drugs can affect your driving, e.g. you may feel drowsy. Until this wears off or you know how your drug affects you, do not drive or operate machinery. You should take extra care, as they may affect your reaction times or reflexes, even though you feel well.

It is an offence to drive, attempt to drive, or to be in charge of a vehicle when unfit through drugs. It is advisable to let your insurance company know if you are taking these drugs. If you do not and you have an accident, it could affect your insurance cover.

What will happen if I stop taking my injection?

If an individual stops taking his injection against the advice of their doctor then the chances of their having another attack are more than doubled. It is, therefore, very important that an individual keeps having their injection even when they feel completely well.

Note: It is worth mentioning at the end about information leaflets, fact sheets and other information available in books and on the Internet.

General tips

When you explain about any medication (antipsychotics, antidepressants, mood stabilizers) make sure that you remember to cover the following important points, which can gain you a global pass!

- Take the medication as directed by the doctor.
- If you are not sure about anything in regard to drugs, such as how many to take or if you have any problems taking your medication, then always ask the pharmacist or doctor.
- Never stop taking your medication without telling your doctor as this can lead to relapse of your illness.

- State the common, less serious side effects first and then mention the serious side effects. State that many side effects will wear off after 2 weeks as your body adjusts to the drugs.

- Some drugs have serious side effects (e.g. lithium, clozapine). Explain these. State that: You must call (doctor, pharmacist or NHS) for help immediately if you think you are suffering any of these side effects.

- Explain if there are special precautions such as blood tests or dietary restrictions associated with the drugs.

- Do not drink alcohol while you are taking medication.

- Do not drive at least for 2 weeks after starting any medication or for 2 weeks after an increase in the dose.

COGNITIVE BEHAVIOURAL THERAPY

Task: Mrs Doherty, a 30-year-old woman suffers from recurrent depressive disorder and shows only partial response to two different antidepressant drugs. You are planning to refer her for CBT. The patient wants to know more about CBT.

Suggested approach

- Greet the patient and introduce yourself.
- Explain the purpose of the visit.
- Obtain permission before you proceed.
- First explain to the patient about your plan to refer her for CBT.

What does CBT stand for?

CBT stands for cognitive behavioural therapy.

What is cognitive therapy?

There are two main types of treatments for depression. One is the physical treatment such as medication or ECT, and the other is the psychological or talking treatments. CBT is one of the most commonly used psychological treatments.

Can you tell me more about it please?

Cognitive therapy is a way of helping people to cope with stress and emotional problems. The idea behind it is quite simple – 'the way we think about things affects how we feel emotionally'.

When people are depressed, they often have negative thoughts about themselves, their future and the world in general. These thoughts come automatically into their minds. These negative thoughts or 'cognitions', undermine their self-confidence, and make them feel even more depressed, leading to unhelpful behaviours. The therapist will work with you to identify the thinking and behavioural patterns that contribute to how you feel, and help you to make changes.

Is it the same as counselling?

CBT is a lot different from counselling. They are both talking treatments, although CBT is much more structured. Counselling is a way of talking through your problems with a counsellor, who can help by listening to your problems. A counsellor may also help you to get a more helpful perspective on problems in your daily life.

How does it work?

Cognitive therapy is a way of talking about the connections between how we think, how we feel and how we behave. It particularly concentrates on ideas that are unrealistic. These often undermine our self-confidence and make us feel depressed or anxious. Looking at these negative thoughts and challenging these negative thoughts can help us work out different ways of thinking and behaving that in turn will help us cope better.

Will I have to lie on a couch and talk about childhood?

Not really. CBT looks at 'here and now' issues rather than things from the past. It helps people to learn new methods of coping and solving problems, which they can use for the rest of their lives.

What is the duration of this therapy?

CBT usually lasts for 8–12 weeks. Usually there will be one session a week, each lasting about 50 minutes.

Who will be seeing me?

Someone with special training and experience in CBT such as a psychologist, a nurse therapist, a psychiatric social worker or a psychiatrist will be seeing you.

What does a course of therapy involve?

In the first few sessions, the client and the therapist decide which problems seem to be the most important. Clients/patients take an active part and carry out 'homework' tasks between sessions. They will often be asked to keep a diary of their thoughts, feelings and behaviours in the situations that they find particularly stressful. They then discuss these in detail in the sessions with the therapists, asking themselves whether or not their ways of thinking are realistic. They can then learn to change these ways of thinking to use more helpful ones.

Whom can it help?

Research has shown that it is particularly helpful for people who suffer from anxiety or depression. It may also be used to treat panic attacks and eating disorders such as bulimia.

Can you have CBT when you are taking antidepressants?

Yes, you can. In fact, the scientific and research evidence is that CBT and antidepressants enhance each other's effects. You can still continue taking your medications and you will still have access to supports like your GP.

Is it useful for anxiety-related problems?

More often depression and anxiety go hand in hand. CBT particularly suits people who want to be actively involved in dealing with their problems. We use CBT techniques to treat both depression and anxiety.

Can CBT prevent depression coming back?

Yes it can. CBT helps by changing your thinking and behaviour patterns and in fact, the last few sessions focus on 'relapse prevention'. Hence, it is effective in reducing the chances of relapse.

But eventually it will be you sorting out your own problems with the help of the CBT therapist. This will need to happen over the long term. You may need to come in from time to time for check-up sessions.

What do I do in an emergency or crisis?

In an emergency or crisis, you will need to use your normal network of support. This could include family, friends and your GP in the first instance, but also other agencies like the crisis intervention team – depending on what you need at the time.

Can I stop if I feel it's not working?

It is always possible to leave therapy, though the pressure to remain may seem stressful at times. Talk about your difficulties with your therapist before you decide to stay or leave. Ultimately, if you want to stop, it is up to you.

■ **It is worth mentioning at the end about information leaflets, fact sheets and other information available in books and on the Internet.**

OBSESSIVE–COMPULSIVE DISORDER AND TREATMENT OPTIONS

Task: Mrs Wilkinson has been diagnosed as suffering from obsessive–compulsive disorder. She wants to know more about the illness and the treatments available. Address her concerns and allay her anxiety.

Suggested approach

- Greet the patient and introduce yourself.

- Explain the purpose of the visit.

- Obtain permission before you proceed.

- Address the patient's main concerns first.

Questions

What is obsessive–compulsive disorder?

Obsessive–compulsive disorder (OCD) is based around obsessive (engrossing) thoughts, for example fear of contamination, as well as a compulsion (urge) to carry out physical rituals such as excessive washing. The ritual behaviour often helps to relieve the fear created by the obsessive thoughts.

People with OCD are usually aware that their obsessive thoughts are irrational, but nevertheless feel powerless to control them.

The compulsions, such as excessive hand washing, are time consuming and can interfere with all aspects of your life – your daily routine, work, and relationships with others, but if the compulsion is not performed, that too creates great anxiety.

How common is this condition?

OCD affects between one to two people in 100 and usually begins in late childhood or adolescence.

Some of the most common obsessions are:

- Worrying about contamination with dirt or germs

- Being overly concerned about symmetry or orderly arrangement of things

- Worrying about unusual sexual thoughts

- Aggressive impulses

- Doubting about things you know you shouldn't worry about.

161

Some of the most common compulsions are:

- Checking
- Washing
- Hoarding
- Counting
- Need to ask or confess.

What causes OCD?

There are several ideas about the causes of OCD:

- One idea is that it is a 'learned' behaviour, in which the person comes to recognize the performance of rituals with relief from anxiety – thus reinforcing the behaviour.

- Another idea says that OCD has a genetic cause – that is, it runs in families. It is known that 25% of people with OCD also have a close relative with the disorder.

- Thirdly, there is an idea that OCD results from changes in the balance of chemicals in the brain. It has been known for some time that one of these chemicals, serotonin, is important in depression – depressed people have low levels of serotonin. It is now also believed that low levels of serotonin are an important factor in people with OCD.

There is in fact a strong link between OCD and depression – two-thirds of people with OCD will be depressed at some point in their lives. One-third will have a major depression when they are first diagnosed as having OCD. It is therefore important to have any depression treated, in addition to the OCD itself.

How is OCD treated?

OCD can be treated through drug treatment, psychological or talking treatment – or by a combination of both.

Drug treatment

The antidepressant medications have been shown to be helpful in treating OCD. As with all medicines, you may find that your drug treatment has some side effects, but these may last only for a short period of time.

The most common side effects found with antidepressant medicines are nausea, headaches, dry mouth, blurred vision, dizziness and feeling sleepy. However it is important to remember that they are not addictive. They will not cause withdrawal symptoms when you stop taking them.

If you are concerned about side effects, which are severe or last for a long time, go back and see your doctor. Your doctor may be able to change your medicine or the dosage.

How long should I take the medications?

If you are given drug treatment for OCD, you may have to stay on treatment for a long time. This is to make sure there's no chance of symptoms returning.

You may find it takes a few weeks for your drugs to start working – your doctor can tell you how soon you can expect to see results. Whatever medicine you're taking, it is important that you keep taking it until your doctor tells you to stop.

What are the psychological or talking treatments that are available?

There are different forms of psychological treatments and the most commonly used treatments are:

1. Exposure and response prevention

2. Cognitive behavioural therapy.

Can you tell me more in detail about exposure and response prevention please?

The treatment strategy involves exposing the individual to stimuli that trigger anxiety or discomfort, and then having the individual voluntarily refrain from performing his or her ritual or compulsion. For each ritual the individual will be required to list a range of situations that cause anxiety and which trigger the urge to perform that ritual.

The individual would then rate each of these situations according to the amount of anxiety or distress that would arise if he or she did not perform the particular ritual.

These are then arranged in order according to those that generate the *least* anxiety or discomfort to those that generate the most anxiety or discomfort. The first task in the list would be an activity that is mildly discomforting but not too difficult, while the last task in the list would be the most difficult task that the individual can imagine.

Answers

Let me explain the steps involved in exposure and response prevention

Step 1: Firstly, provide training for slow breathing exercises and relaxation. These exercises can be used prior to commencing each step of the graded exposure hierarchy to ensure that the individual is calm and relatively relaxed at the beginning of each graded exposure session.

Step 2: Identify a first small step towards overcoming the feared ritual.

Step 3: Practise this step until it no longer causes anxiety.

Step 4: Move on to a more difficult step and repeat the practise.

Step 5: Continue this process until the person can manage the last step towards overcoming the ritual.

It is worth mentioning the following points:

- This is a simple but highly effective technique.

- It is usually done in graded steps.

- The active participation of clients is necessary.

- The situation can be real or imagined (a real-life situation will be more effective).

- It can be practised regularly with self-exposure tasks.

- It is used particularly in treatment of phobias and OCD.

Cognitive behavioural therapy

See previous chapters for CBT explanation.

What will happen in the future?

It may seem difficult to believe right now, but with the right treatment it is possible for most people to overcome an OCD. Progress may be slow, but complete recovery is possible. Remember to follow your doctor's advice; including taking any medicine you are given every day.

- **It is worth mentioning at the end about information leaflets, fact sheets and other information available in books and on the Internet.**

TREATMENT OPTIONS FOR AGORAPHOBIA

Task: Mrs Brown is a 47-year-old woman who lives with her husband. She suffers from agoraphobia. She has come to see you to discuss the treatment options available. Address her concerns and allay her anxiety.

Suggested approach

- Greet the patient and introduce yourself.

- Explain the purpose of the visit.

- Obtain permission before you proceed.

- Address the patient's main concerns first.

Treatment options

What are the treatment options available for agoraphobia?

Agoraphobia is a common problem and it is definitely treatable. There are a number of different treatments available including education, psychological treatments and medication.

Education may sound simple, but you and your family need to know about the nature of the illness, what keeps it going and how to deal with it.

What are the medications available for treatment of agoraphobia?

There are two main types of medication: benzodiazepines and antidepressants. Benzodiazepines for example (Valium) start working very quickly and can be useful in the short term but they are addictive, and you may become dependent on them. However, antidepressants would be a very good option.

Does that mean that I am depressed?

No, not at all. Even though they are called antidepressants, these drugs are useful to treat a variety of conditions like depression, anxiety, panic attacks and agoraphobias. They treat and modify the chemical imbalance in the brain that is common to all these disorders.

How do you go about it?

We start them at a low dose and increase gradually. They may take up to 8 weeks to start working. Once you feel better, you will have to continue the medication for about 6 months, if not longer. Then we have to taper it off gradually and stop. They are not addictive.

What about psychological treatments?

The name of the psychological treatment offered is called 'systematic desensitisation'.

Systematic desensitisation

This treatment is also called 'graded exposure with relaxation'. In this therapy, first we will teach you relaxation exercises to help you control your anxiety and panic. Then we make a list of hierarchy of situations that you find difficult to face. We arrange them from the least difficult to the most difficult.

Then you start by facing the easiest situation, whilst managing to relax. When you feel comfortable with that situation, you then go onto the next one. You will have to practise this daily.

You may find it easier to face situations if you move from the least difficult to the most difficult, e.g. like going out of the front door of your house, going out to your garden from your house, then going out to a nearby shop with a family member/friend and then going out to a supermarket with a family member/friend and so on. Practise the steps until it no longer causes anxiety. Move on to a more difficult step and repeat the practise.

I can't come out of my house, as I am worried that I might collapse. How can you help me in this situation?

We can understand your difficulties. In that case, we can arrange for the therapist to come to your house to help you initially.

You mentioned my family members; what can they do?

Your family members and/or your partner have an important role in the treatment process. It would be very helpful if they also learn how the therapy works, so that they are able to support, motivate and help you to tackle problems that keep the illness going. They could support you and accompany you for the treatment sessions, so it will be very helpful if they can also be involved.

- It is worth mentioning at the end about information leaflets, fact sheets and other information available in books and on the Internet.

PANIC DISORDER AND HYPERVENTILATION SYNDROME

Task: Mr Williams is a 48-year-old man who suffers from a panic disorder. His father recently died of a heart attack and there is a strong family history of ischaemic heart disease. He is therefore concerned that he might suffer from heart attacks. Address his concerns and explain to him about how hyperventilation can worsen panic attacks.

Suggested approach

- Greet the patient and introduce yourself.

- Explain the purpose of the visit.

- Obtain permission before you proceed.

- Address the patient's main concerns first.

- Reassure the patient that he is not having a heart attack and it is only a panic attack.

Reassurance

You can reassure the patient by saying that:

- A person with a panic attack might think that he or she is having a heart attack. This is because some of the symptoms of a panic attack are also experienced during a heart attack, for example chest pain and breathlessness. It is therefore understandable that a person who is having a panic attack may think he or she is having a heart attack. If chest pain is recurrent or long lasting, it is wise to have a thorough medical investigation to rule out the presence of heart disease. If heart disease is not present then it is unlikely that subsequent chest pain is caused by a heart attack.

- It is probably best for him or her to sit quietly and use the slow breathing exercise for about 5–10 minutes. However, if pain is still present after 10 minutes of slow breathing, the individual is advised to seek medical advice.

What happens during a panic attack and when does this occur?

Panic disorder involves recurrent and sometimes unpredictable attacks of anxiety or panic. The attacks start suddenly without any obvious precipitants, are extremely distressing, and last for a few minutes, sometimes longer. In panic disorder the attacks are not restricted to specific circumstances but may occur in any situation.

Panic attacks are defined by a sudden onset of intense apprehension, fear of dying, losing control or going mad accompanied by physical symptoms such as difficulty in breathing, dizziness, palpitations, chest pains, shaking, sweating and tingling sensations.

During a panic attack individuals will generally try to flee from the particular situation in the hope that the panic will stop and relieve their anxiety, or else they may seek help in case they collapse, have a heart attack, or go crazy.

These attacks may be followed by persistent concern about having another panic attack and can make the patient feel more anxious.

What is the panic response?

When we are exposed to a physical threat, our bodies automatically respond so that we are able to defend ourselves or escape from a threatening situation. This response is also known as the 'flight-or-fight' response. As a result of this, our body prepares itself to run away or fight and therefore we become more alert, our heart beat speeds up, the muscles get tense and sweating increases to cool the body, and we breathe very fast in order to get more oxygen to our muscles.

Consequently we breathe out carbon dioxide; this makes the level in our body low and produces strange physical sensations like dizziness, tingling in our hands and feet, pains in the chest and breathlessness. When people feel breathless, they breathe faster and this will make your symptoms worse.

It is important to realize that these feelings are part of the physical response to threat and are not a sign that you have some physical disease. These symptoms do not mean that you will die, go crazy, or lose control. However, because they are part of a stress response, it may be useful for you to look at your life and try to identify what might be troubling you and adding to your stress at the moment.

What happens during hyperventilation?

When you become anxious and panicky it leads to an increase in the speed and depth of breathing. This over-breathing, also called 'hyperventilation', may lead to the following symptoms:

- In the brain it causes dizziness, light-headedness, confusion, breathlessness, and feelings of unreality. In the body it causes an increase in heartbeat, numbness and tingling in the hands and feet, cold clammy hands, stiffness in the muscles, muscle twitching or cramps and irregular heartbeats.

- People who over-breathe often tend to breathe from their chest rather than from their diaphragm. As the chest muscles are not made for breathing, these muscles tend to become tired and tense. Thus individuals can experience symptoms of chest tightness or even severe chest pains.

How can we prevent and control hyperventilation?

The first step in preventing and controlling hyperventilation is to recognize *how* and *when* hyperventilation occurs.

In order to reduce the symptoms of hyperventilation it will be necessary to increase and steady the level of carbon dioxide in the blood, which will help the individual reduce habitual over-breathing. This is done by practising the slow breathing exercise.

Here the individual is instructed to *breathe in* and hold his or her breath, and then instructed to breathe slowly out, saying the word relax to themselves in a calm, soothing manner every time they breathe out. This should be repeated in cycles until all the symptoms of over-breathing have gone.

If individuals follow this exercise as soon as they notice the first signs of over-breathing, the symptoms should subside within a minute or two and panic attacks will hopefully be avoided. The more frequently individuals practise this slow breathing exercise, the better they will become at using slow breathing to prevent anxiety from escalating.

What to do next?

It is very likely that you will be more able to manage panic attacks in the future if:

● You recognize that the symptoms are harmless and understand the mechanism of fight-or-flight response.

● You remember to use the slow breathing exercise when you get anxious

● You learn how to relax and manage your stress more effectively.

■ It is worth mentioning at the end about information leaflets, fact sheets and other information available in books and on the Internet.

Examinations

MINI-MENTAL STATE EXAMINATION

Task: Perform the MMSE on Mr White, an elderly person who presented himself to the A&E department in a confused state.

Points to be covered

- Temporal orientation
- Spatial orientation
- Registration
- Attention, concentration
- Recall
- Naming
- Repetition
- Comprehension
- Reading
- Writing
- Drawing/copying.

Suggested approach

- Greet the patient and introduce yourself.
- Explain the purpose of the visit.
- Obtain permission before you proceed.
- Address whether there are any major concerns.
- Check the patient's ability to hear, see and understand you.

Max. score	Score	
		Orientation
5	( )	'What is the (year), (season), (month), (date), (day)?'
5	( )	'Where are we?': (country, county, city/town, building name, floor of the building)
		Registration
3	( )	Ask if you can test the individual's memory. Name three objects (e.g. apple, table, penny) taking 1 second to say each one. Then ask the individual to repeat the names of

all three objects. Give one point for each correct answer. After this, repeat the object names until all three are learned – up to six trials).

Attention and calculation

5 ( ) Spell 'world' backwards. Give 1 point for each letter that is in the right order DLROW = 5, DLORW = 3).

Alternatively, do serial 7s. Ask the individual to count backwards from 100 in blocks of 7 (93, 86, 79, 72, 65). 'Now I would like you to take 7 away from 100. Now take away from the number you get. Now keep subtracting until I tell you to stop'. Stop after 5 subtractions. Give one point for each correct answer. If one answer is incorrect (e.g. 92) but the following answer is 7 less than the previous answer (i.e. 85), count the second answer as being correct.

Recall

3 ( ) Ask for the three objects repeated above. 'What were the three objects I asked you to repeat a little while ago?' Give 1 point for each correct object. (Recall should be tested 5 minutes after presenting the words).

Language

2 ( ) Point to a pencil and ask the individual to name this object (1 point).

Do the same with a wrist-watch (1 point).

1 ( ) Ask the individual to repeat the following: 'No ifs, ands or buts' (1 point).

You may repeat the phrase if the individual has difficulty hearing or understanding you, up to a maximum of five times, but the score should be based only on the first attempt to repeat the phrase.

3 ( ) Give the individual a piece of blank white paper and ask him or her to follow a three-stage command. 'Take the paper in your right hand, fold it in half with both hands and put the paper down on your lap' (1 point for each part correctly followed). Give only one trial.

1 ( ) Show the individual the 'CLOSE YOUR EYES' message. Ask him or her to read the message and do what it says (give 1 point if the individual actually closes his or her eyes).

1 ( ) Ask the individual to write a sentence on a blank piece of paper. The sentence must contain a subject (real or implied) and a verb, and must be sensible. Punctuation and grammar are not important (1 point).

1 ( ) Show the individual the intersecting pentagons and ask him or her to copy the design exactly as it is (1 point). Each

pentagon should have five sides and five clear corners and the two shapes must intersect to score 1 point. Tremor and rotation are ignored.

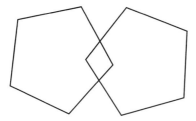

Total score = ...

■ Thank the patient for their co-operation.

PERFORM DETAILED COGNITIVE EXAMINATION

Task: Perform cognitive examination on Mr Black, an elderly person who presented himself to the A&E department in a confused state.

This can be asked as a complex CASC station as there are many tasks to be covered.

Detailed cognitive assessment involve checking for:

- Orientation to time, place and person
- Attention and concentration
- Calculation
- Memory – working memory, anterograde and retrograde memory
- Language
- Visuospatial and visuoconstructive functions
- Executive functions
- Assessment of praxis.

Orientation to time, place and person

- Orientation to time:
  a. 'What is the year?'
  b. 'What is the season?'
  c. 'What is the month?'
  d. 'What is the day of the week?'
  e. 'What is the date?'
- Orientation to place
  a. 'What is the country?'
  b. 'What is the county/state/province?'
  c. 'Which city are we in?'
  d. 'What is the name of the hospital or building?'
  e. 'Which floor are we on?'
- Orientation to person
  a. 'Can you please tell me your full name?'
  b. 'How old are you?'
  c. 'What is your occupation?'

Attention and concentration

Serial reversal tasks include spelling W-O-R-L-D backwards, serial 7s from 100. The other tests include reciting months of the year backwards, and the days of the week backwards.

Calculations

Ask the patient to perform mental arithmetic such as additions, subtraction, multiplication or division. For example ask the patient to write down four or five numbers and add them up.

Memory

Working memory:

Forward digit span: Here a series of numbers is read to the subject, who then repeats the numbers back. The numbers should be read evenly at one per second and start from three digits. The normal range is 6+/−1.
Backward digit span: Here the subject is asked to repeat the string of numbers backwards (e.g. the examiner reads 396 and the patient reads 693). The normal range is 5+/−1.

Anterograde memory (new learning)

Registration and recall of three items

Ask if you can test the individual's memory. Name three objects (e.g. apple, table, penny) taking 1 second to say each one. Then ask the individual to repeat the names of all three objects.

Ask for the three objects repeated earlier. What were the three objects I asked you to repeat a little while ago? Give 1 point for each correct object. (Recall should be tested 5 minutes after presenting the words).

Registration and recall of a seven-item name and address

I am going to read you a name and address that I would like you to repeat after me. We will be doing it three times so that you have a chance to learn it and I will be asking you about it later.

Then read out the following address:

John Brown,
42, West Street, Luton
Bedfordshire

This can be recorded as a score out of 7 on the first learning trial, e.g. 4/7. Repeat the entire name and address in completion before the subject again tries to complete. Recall can be tested at 5–10 minutes. A score of 5 or less may give cause for concern if all seven items were learnt.

Retrograde memory (memory for personal events)

- 'Where did you grow up and go to school?'
- 'When did you finish school?'
- 'When did you get married?'

Semantic memory (general events)

- 'Who is the current prime minister of the UK?'
- 'Who is the previous prime minister of the UK?'
- 'Who is the current president of USA?'
- 'Who is the previous president of USA?'
- 'What are the years of the Second World War?'
- 'Did anything important happen in the world on September 11th, 2001?' (description of any recent news events like political, sports events, accidents, catastrophes).

Language

1. Comprehension

Simple commands, e.g. 'Close your eyes, touch your nose.'

2. Repetition: Sentences that are used for testing

- Repeat 'No ifs ands or buts'
- The orchestra played and the audience applauded.

3. Naming

Point to two or three objects and ask patient to name them. Ask the patient to name high-frequency global names such as (e.g. Watch, Jacket) and also more specific/less frequency items such as (e.g Label or Winder) that are generally more difficult.

4. Word fluency

Ask patients to generate a list of as many animals as possible in 1 minute (normal 15 in a category in 1 minute). Typical categories used to test include animals, fruits, vehicles, etc.

5. Reading

Show the individual the 'CLOSE YOUR EYES' message. Ask him or her to read the message.

6. Writing

Ask the individual to write a sentence on a blank piece of paper. The sentence must contain a subject (real or implied) and a verb, and must be sensible.

Visuospatial and visuoconstructive functions

Asking the subject to copy drawings or shapes, which are three-dimensional in nature, tests this.

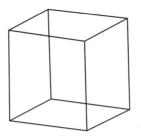

Clock drawing test

Draw a circle and ask the subject to fill in numbers and hands to current time and tell the subject to set the time at 10 to 5.

In this task look for signs of neglect or of disorganization in the approach. This can indicate perceptual and perceptuomotor deficits, constructional apraxia and unilateral neglect.

Executive function

This involves frontal lobe functions that includes verbal fluency, cognitive estimation, abstract thinking and reasoning, response inhibition, motor sequencing and programming (please read chapter on 'frontal lobe function testing').

Praxis

Ideomotor praxis

- 'Show me how you brush your teeth.'

- 'Show me how you comb your hair.'

- 'Show me how you cut paper with scissors.'

Ideational praxis

The subject should be asked to perform a complex task with multiple steps, for example placing a letter in an envelope, sealing it, addressing it, stamping it and then posting it.

Orobuccal praxis

Here the subject is asked to carry out specific movements on command like 'stick out your tongue', 'lick your lips', etc.

■ Thank the patient and the examiner.

FRONTAL LOBE FUNCTION TESTING

Task: Assess the frontal lobe functions for this 65-year-old man with memory problems.

Suggested approach

- Greet the patient and introduce yourself.

- Confirm the identity of the patient.

- Explain briefly what you are going to do and obtain verbal consent from the patient.

Frontal executive function tests

1. Assessment of verbal fluency/category fluency

The patient is asked to name as many words as possible beginning with either the letters 'F, A or S' in 1 minute (ideally all three ought to be tested). Normal subjects should produce at least 15 words for each letter. Less than 10 items is definitely abnormal.

   Alternatively you can use a category (name as many animals as possible in 1 minute). Typical categories used to test include animals, fruits, vehicles etc.

2. Assessment of abstraction

Proverb interpretation

Ask the patient the meaning of two common proverbs:
Example 1: Too many cooks spoil the broth.
Example 2: A stitch in time saves nine.

Similarities

The patient is asked to explain the similarities between things (use things that are routinely used), for example:

a. Table and chair

b. Apple and orange

c. Glass and ice.

3. Cognitive estimation

Ask the patient to make estimates such as:

- 'What is the height of an average Englishman?'

- 'How many camels are there in England?'

4. Co-ordinated movements (tests response inhibition and set shifting)

Alternate sequence
An alternative sequence of squares and triangles are shown to the patient and they are asked to copy it.

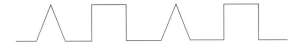

Go-no-go test

Ask the patient to place a hand on the table and to raise one finger in response to a single tap, while holding still in response to two taps. You tap on the under surface of the table to avoid giving visual cues.

Luria three-step task

A sequence of hand positions is demonstrated which would be placing a fist, then edge of the palm and then a flat palm onto the palm of the opposite hand and repeating the sequence (fist-edge-palm). It can be demonstrated up to five times.

5. Frontal lobe release signs

Glabellar tap

Tap between the patients' eyebrows, which causes repeated blinking even after five or more taps, if it is positive.

Primitive reflex

This would include Grasp reflex in which you stroke the patient's palm while distracting the patient; watch for involuntary grasping and pouting reflex when you tap on a spatula on patient's lips, resulting in spouting and both reflexes can be subtle.

■ Thank the patient and the examiner.

PARIETAL LOBE FUNCTION TESTING

Task: Assess the parietal lobe functions for this 65-year-old man with memory problems.

Suggested approach

- Greet the patient and introduce yourself.

- Confirm the identity of the patient.

- Explain briefly what you are going to do and obtain verbal consent from the patient.

Dominant parietal lobe tests

Finger agnosia

Ask the patient to name which finger you touched. Touch at least two fingers on each side.

Right-left disorientation

Ask the patient to put their right hand on the desk, then remove it. Repeat with left hand, then right hand again.

Calculation

Ask the patient to write down four or five numbers and add them up. Ask the patient to perform mental arithmetic such as additions, subtraction, multiplication or division.

Writing

Ask the patient to write a sentence, e.g. 'She went to the store to buy shoes.'

Praxis

Ask the patient to mime how they would clean their teeth, blow out a match, comb their hair, use scissors, etc. Watch their ability to do these and also for use of body parts as objects.

Astereoagnosia

Ask the patient with eyes closed to identify coins in hand or familiar objects.

Dysgraphaesthesia

Ask the patient with eyes closed to recognize letters or numbers written on the hand.

Non-dominant parietal lobe tests

Unilateral neglect

Ask the patient with eyes closed to tell you which hand you touched. Touch left, right and then both together.

Postural arm drift

Ask the patient to hold out the arms, palms down, and eyes closed. Watch for drift of either hand downwards. Arm drift indicates contralateral parietal lobe abnormality.

Constructional apraxia

Show the individual the intersecting pentagons and ask him or her to copy the design exactly as it is. Each pentagon should have five sides and five clear corners and the two shapes must intersect. Please see MMSE for the figure.

- Thank the patient and the examiner.

EXTRAPYRAMIDAL SIDE EFFECTS – PHYSICAL EXAMINATION

Task: Mr Jones has been diagnosed as having paranoid schizophrenia and has been started on one of the conventional antipsychotics. However, he is complaining of stiffness in his arms and legs. Address his concerns and examine him for extrapyramidal signs.

EPSEs would include:

a. Akathisia (motor restlessness)

b. Dystonia (uncontrolled muscular contraction)

c. Pseudoparkinsonism – tremor, rigidity, bradykinesia, mask-like facies and festinant gait

d. Tardive dyskinesia (abnormal movements).

Suggested approach

- Greet the patient and introduce yourself.

- Address the patient's concerns first.

- Ask the patient briefly about any abnormal movements like slowness, stiffness, shakiness, feeling of inner restlessness and any other body movements that bother the patient.

- Explain briefly what you are going to do and ask for consent (obtain permission before you proceed).

- Ensure that the patient knows that during this examination you will be testing his hands, legs, and mouth and that you will make him walk to observe his gait.

- Observe the patient at rest for a few seconds.

- Ask the patient whether there is anything in his or her mouth and, if so, to remove it.

- Ask if he or she wears dentures. Ask whether teeth or dentures bother the patient now.

- Ask whether the patient notices any movements in his or her mouth, face, hands, or feet. If yes, ask the patient to describe them and to indicate to what extent they bother the patient.

- Ask the patient to open his or her mouth (observe the tongue at rest within the mouth.) Do this twice.

- Ask the patient to protrude his or her tongue (observe abnormalities of tongue movement). Do this twice.

- Have the patient sit in chair with hands on knees, legs slightly apart and feet flat on floor. (Look at the entire body for movements while the patient is in this position. Observe for 15 seconds.)

- Ask the patient to sit with hands hanging unsupported – if male, between his legs, if female and wearing a dress, hanging over her knees (observe hands and other body areas for at least 15 seconds).

- Ask the patient to tap his or her thumb with each finger as rapidly as possible for 10–15 seconds, first with right hand, then with left hand. (Observe facial, hand and leg movements.)

- Flex and extend the patient's left and right arms, one at a time.

- Ask the patient to stand up. (Observe the patient [for 15 seconds]. Observe all body areas again, hip included.)

- Ask the patient to extend both arms out in front, palms down. (Observe trunk, legs, and mouth.)

- Have the patient walk a few paces, turn, and walk back to the chair. (Observe hands and gait.) Do this twice.

- Give a brief report of your findings and thank the patient and the examiner.

CRANIAL NERVES

Task: Examine cranial nerves 1–12 on this patient except for testing of the corneal reflex and fundoscopy.

Suggested approach

- Greet the patient and introduce yourself.
- Explain the purpose of the visit.
- Obtain permission before you proceed.
- Address any major concerns expressed.
- Take a brief history of sight, smell, taste and hearing.

1st cranial nerve

(Usually questioning is all that is required unless equipment is provided to check formally)

- 'Do you have difficulty with your sense of smell?'
- 'Did you smell your coffee this morning?'

2nd cranial nerve

To check for visual acuity:

- 'Do you have any difficulty with your vision?'
- Sit in front of the patient. (If he has glasses for long sight he should put them on).

    a. Check one eye at a time by asking to close other eye. Do the test by finger counting method.

    or

    b. A near vision chart is provided. Ask the patient to read sections of print from a distance of 30 cm. The smallest size that can be read is recorded (e.g. N6).

To check for field of vision:

- **Mapping visual fields:** Be at the same eye level with the patient. Ask the patient to cover their right eye with their right hand, and cover your left eye with your left hand, and then ask the patient to look in your eye without moving their head. Move your finger to check peripheral fields.

Colour vision:

Not essential.

Pupils

- **Direct and consensual reflexes:** A bright light is shone into one eye and the reaction of both pupils (direct and consensual reflexes) is noted. Before you flash the light make sure you tell the patient that you will be shining a bright light in his eyes, which may cause a bit of discomfort.

- **Accommodation reflex:** The patient is asked to look into the distance and then at a finger positioned 10 cm directly in front of his/her nose. The pupils are examined as the patient attempts to focus on the finger and the reaction of the pupils to accommodation are noted.

Tell the examiner that ideally you would like to perform fundoscopy to examine the optic disc.

3rd, 4th and 6th nerves

Ask the patient to look into your eyes and to follow your moving finger without moving his head. Describe the letter H with your finger, beginning at the centre of the horizontal line, go to left then up and down, bring the finger back to opposite side and do the same. The patient is asked to report any double vision. Watch for nystagmus.

5th cranial nerve

Sensory part

Check superficial sensation on various parts of the face with a cotton swab in all three dermatomes alternating both sides. Ask the patient to close his eyes before you proceed and to answer 'Yes' when he feels the swab.

Motor part

- Check the muscles of mastication.

- Ask the patient to clench the teeth, then feel for the masseters and temporalis.

- Ask the patient to open the mouth against resistance from your hand, which should be placed firmly under the patient's chin.

- You have been asked to ignore the jaw jerk and corneal reflexes.

7th cranial nerve

Sensory part

- 'Did you *taste* your breakfast this morning?'

Motor part

- 'Can you show me your teeth please?'

- Ask him to shut his eyes tightly while you try to open them gently – 'Screw your eyes up tight'.

- Other tests: Ask the patient to raise his eyebrows, blow out his cheeks, and purse his lips tightly.

8th cranial nerve (vestibulocochlear)

- Check whether there is any problem with the hearing in either ear.

- Test hearing sensitivity to a whispered sound or a ticking wristwatch. Alternatively rub finger and thumb together in front of each ear in turn and ask whether the patient can hear that.

- If there is no problem in hearing inform the patient that you'd like to conduct detailed hearing tests, once you've tested the other nerves.

9th and 10th cranial nerves

- Request the patient opens his mouth and ask him to say 'AAAHHH' loudly; comment on soft palate and uvulary movement.

- You have been asked to ignore the gag reflex.

11th cranial nerve

- Ask the patient to shrug shoulders against resistance: 'Shrug your shoulders and keep them shrugged' (push down on the shoulders).

- Ask the patient to turn his head in both directions against resistance: 'Turn your head to the left side, now to the right' (feel for the sternomastoid muscle on the side opposite to the turned head).

12th cranial nerve

- Ask the patient to open his mouth and show his tongue and look for any deviation, wasting or tremors.

- Inspect the tongue as it lies on the floor of the mouth, noting any wasting, fasciculation and involuntary movement.

- Then ask the patient to stick out the tongue and waggle it from side to side.

■ State whether the examination is normal or not and what you would be doing next.

■ Thank the patient and the examiner.

THYROID GLAND

Task: Mrs Smith suffers from bipolar affective disorder. She is currently on lithium 800 mg and over the last 6 months she has been feeling increasingly tired and lethargic. Carry out an examination to assess the patient for thyroid disorder.

Suggested approach

Examination of thyroid gland

- Greet the patient and introduce yourself.
- Explain the purpose of the visit.
- Obtain permission before you proceed.
- Build a rapport and address the patient's main concerns.
- In the case of a female patient, ask for a chaperone.

General examination

- Nails – look for pallor/clubbing/cyanosis
- Hands – sweating/warmth/acropachy/acrocyanosis
- Tremors: Ask the patient to stretch out his hands for full extension of the wrist and elbow. If the tremor is not obvious, place your palm against the patient's outstretched fingers to feel for it. Alternatively, you can place a piece of paper on the dorsum of the patient's outstretched hands and it will oscillate if a fine tremor is present.
- Pulse – rate and rhythm
- Tongue – pallor/cyanosis
- Legs – pretibial myxoedema.

Local examination

Check the exposure from the jaw to the nipple line.

Inspection

Pizzillo's method: The patient's hands are placed behind the head and the head is pushed backwards against the clasped hands. Look for:

- Any obvious swelling on swallowing and on protrusion of tongue: the thyroid swelling usually moves upwards on swallowing
- Sinuses and erythema
- Any dilated or engorged veins in the neck and on the chest
- Visible pulsations, if any.

Palpation (from front)

- Confirm findings of inspection

- Feel for the trachea and its displacement, if present

- Carotid pulsations: feel one at a time

- The thyroid gland should ideally be palpated with the patient's neck slightly flexed. The gland may be palpated from behind and from the front with the four fingers of each hand placed on each lobe.

- Lower limit of thyroid is checked while the patient is swallowing

- Check for cervical lymphadenopathy.

Percussion

- Only if lower limit of the gland is not palpable (direct percussion on the sternum).

Auscultation

- Check for thyroid and carotid bruit.

Eye signs

- *Exophthalmos (from behind):* Relative protrusion of the eyes can be observed by standing behind a seated patient and looking downward toward the chin from the forehead to assess the displacement of one globe as compared to the contralateral side. The patient should also be examined from the side.

- *Check for lid lag:* Hold the patient's head still with one hand and ask her to follow the index finger of the other hand. Move it up and then down. With lid lag, as the finger moves down, some white cornea is seen above the iris.

Reflexes

- *Ankle jerk:* The slow relaxing ankle jerk is usually best demonstrated with the patient kneeling on a chair or bed with the feet hanging over the edge, and the examiner standing behind the patient.

- Ask the patient to dress.

- Thank the patient and the examiner.

Clinical symptoms of hyperthyroidism

Symptoms

- Weight loss despite increased appetite

- Heat intolerance, sweating, diarrhoea

- Tremors
- Irritability, anxiety
- Oligomenorrhoea, infertility.

Signs

- Tachycardia, atrial fibrillation
- Warm extremities, palmar erythema
- Fine tremors
- Goitre and nodules
- Hair thinning
- Lid lag, lid retraction, exophthalmos.

Clinical symptoms of hypothyroidism

Symptoms

- Tiredness, lethargy, myalgia
- Weight gain
- Constipation
- Dislike of cold
- Menorrhagia
- Hoarse voice
- Depression, dementia.

Signs

- Bradycardia
- Dry skin and hair
- Goitre
- Slowly relaxing reflexes
- Congestive cardiac failure, non-pitting oedema, pericardial effusion
- Toad-like face
- Peripheral neuropathy.

SENSORY AND MOTOR EXAMINATION OF UPPER LIMBS

Task: Perform sensory and motor system examination of upper limbs for this 49-year-old man admitted recently to your ward.

Suggested approach

- Introduce yourself to the patient.
- Confirm the identity of the patient.
- Obtain verbal consent from the patient.
- Ensure privacy and achieve adequate exposure.
- In case of females, do not forget to ask for a chaperone.
- Ask the relevant neurological history such as history of tingling, numbness, heaviness, etc.
- Uncover the limb to be examined with the consent of the patient.

General examination

- Nails – pallor, cyanosis, capillary filling and trophic changes
- Hair loss on the limb
- Any obvious joint pathology
- Pulse.

Inspection

- Posture of limb
- Look for any obvious deformity
- Wasting of limb and fasciculation
- Scars, sinuses, erythema or swelling.

Palpation

- Ask permission before you proceed
- Temperature – compare both sides
- Limb girth measurement – above and below the joint.

Sensory examination

For this exam purpose you check for:

Dorsal column

Superficial sensation
Test using a cotton swab. The patient should have his eyes closed. The patient should feel the cotton swab on his face or sternum before you proceed.

Vibration sense
Use a 128 Hz frequency tuning fork. Tell patient that this is a tuning fork and when you place it on his bony prominences it will feel like a buzz. Usually it is tested on the first metacarpo-phalangeal joint for an upper limb. Here again make the patient feel the tuning fork on his sternum before you proceed and ensure his eyes are closed.

Positional sense
Tested by checking movement of the distal interphalangeal joint of the thumb with eyes closed. If the patient cannot feel the position then check the proximal joints till he feels it. (If he cannot feel moving first distal interphalangeal joint, then move the wrist; if still negative, move the elbow joint.)

Lateral column

Pain sensation
Tested here with red-headed pins on the dermatomes. They do not usually allow the pain sensation to be tested, but you must mention that ideally you would like to test it.

Temperature
Mention that ideally you would like to test the temperature also.

Motor examination

Check for the muscle bulk on both the sides in the upper arms, lower arms and hands.

Check for tone: Ensure that he does not have any joint pain in that limb. Test the tone in the arms by passively bending the arm to and fro and in the hands by flexing and extending all the joints, including the wrist.

Check power

Put your arms out to the side with arms at 90 degrees to your body with elbows flexed (best to demonstrate this to the patient yourself).

- Deltoid (C-5) – 'Stop me pushing them down.'

- Biceps (C-5,6) – 'Bend your elbow, stop me straightening it.'

- Triceps (C-7) – 'Push your arm out straight and resist elbow extension.'

- Offer two fingers and ask the patient to squeeze your fingers (C-8, T-1).

- Spread your fingers apart and stop me pushing them together (dorsal interossei-ulnar nerve).

- Hold this piece of paper between your fingers; stop me pulling it out (palmar interossei-ulnar nerve).

Reflexes

- Check for biceps C5, C6.

- Check for triceps C7.

- Check for supinator C5, C6.

Cerebellar signs

- Upper limb: finger–nose test (one test is enough) – touch my finger, touch your nose; backwards and forwards quickly and neatly

- Check for involuntary movements – tremor (fasciculation).

Conclusion

- For upper limbs – mention examination of cervical spine.

- Make sure the patient is dressed.

- Thank the patient and the examiner.

SENSORY AND MOTOR EXAMINATION OF LOWER LIMBS

Task: Perform sensory and motor system examination of lower limbs for this 42-year-old man admitted recently to your ward.

Suggested approach

- Introduce yourself to the patient.
- Confirm the identity of the patient.
- Obtain verbal consent from the patient.
- Ensure privacy and achieve adequate exposure.
- In case of females, do not forget to ask for a chaperone.
- Ask the relevant neurological history such as history of tingling, numbness, heaviness, etc.
- Uncover the limb to be examined with the consent of the patient.

General examination

- Nails – pallor, cyanosis, capillary filling and trophic changes
- Hair loss on the limb
- Any obvious joint pathology
- Pulse.

Inspection

- Posture of limb
- Look for any obvious deformity
- Wasting of limb and fasciculation
- Scars, sinuses, erythema or swelling.

Palpation

- Ask permission before you proceed
- Temperature – compare both sides
- Limb girth measurement – above and below the joint.

Sensory examination

For this exam purpose you check for:

Dorsal column

Superficial sensation

Test using a cotton swab. The patient should have his eyes closed. The patient should feel the cotton swab on his face or sternum before you proceed.

Vibration sense

Use a 128 Hz frequency tuning fork. Tell patient that this is a tuning fork and when you place it on his bony prominences it will feel like a buzz. Usually it is tested on the first metatarso-phalangeal joint or on the medial malleoli for the lower limbs. Here again make the patient feel the tuning fork on his sternum before you proceed and ensure his eyes are closed.

Positional sense

Tested by checking movement of the distal interphalangeal joint of the big toe with eyes closed. If the patient cannot feel the position then check the proximal joints until he feels it. (If he cannot feel moving the first distal interphalangeal joint, then move the ankle; if the response is still negative, move the knee joint.)

Lateral column

Pain sensation

Tested here with red-headed pins on the dermatomes. They do not usually allow the pain sensation to be tested, but you must mention that ideally you would like to test it.

Temperature

Mention that ideally you would like to test the temperature also.

Motor examination

Muscle bulk

Check for muscle bulk above and below the knee joint.

Tone

Ensure that he does not have any joint pain in that limb. Examine the muscle tone in each leg by passively moving it at the hip and knee joints – roll the leg sideways, backwards and forwards on the bed, lift the knee and let it drop or bend the knee.

Power

- Tell the patient to lift their leg up and ask the patient to stop you pushing it down (L1,2).

- Tell the patient to bend their knee and don't let me straighten it (L5, S1,2).

- With knee still bent, tell the patient to push their leg out straight against my hand (L3,4).

- Tell the patient to bend their foot down and push my hand away (S1).

- Tell the patient to cock up their foot, point their toes at the ceiling and stop me pushing the foot down (L4,5).

Reflexes

- Check for knee reflexes (L3,4).

- Check for ankle jerks (S1,2) and check for ankle clonus at the same time.

- Check the plantar reflex.

Cerebellar signs

- Knee–heel test: Tell the patient to 'put your heel just below your knee then run it smoothly down your shin, now up your shin, now down' etc.

- Romberg's test: This should be tested with the patient's feet together and the arms outstretched. Make sure that you are ready to catch the patient if there is any possibility of ataxia.

- Check for gait, and involuntary movements.

Conclusion

- Ideally mention that you will also examine the dorsolumbar spine.

- Make sure the patient is dressed.

- Thank the patient and the examiner.

CARDIOVASCULAR

Task: Examine the cardiovascular system of this 44-year-old man admitted to your ward.

Suggested approach

- Introduce yourself to the patient.
- Confirm the identity of the patient.
- Obtain verbal consent from the patient.
- Ensure privacy and achieve adequate exposure.
- In case of females, do not forget to ask for a chaperone.

General examination

Observe whether the patient is breathless, cyanosed, and pale or whether he/she has a 'malar' flush (on the face):

- **Eyes** – Jaundice and pallor
- **Tongue** – Pallor and cyanosis
- **Nails** – Pallor/clubbing/cyanosis/splinter haemorrhage
- **Palm** – Palmar erythema
- **Pulse** – Rate and rhythm with radial pulse. Volume and character in brachial pulses on both sides
- **Carotids** – Check one at a time
- **JVP** – Ask the patient to recline at an angle of 45 degrees on the couch. Turn his head to the left side and look for any rise of JVP
- **Oedema** – Ankles, but mention that you would like to look for sacral oedema.

Systemic examination

Inspection

- Apex beat: localize the apex beat with respect to the mid-clavicular line and rib spaces, firstly by inspection for visible pulsation
- Deformity
- Redness, scars and sinuses
- Engorged veins.

Palpation

Remember to ask for permission before touching the patient:

- **Locate the apex beat and mention its character:** If the apex beat is rigorous, then you should be able to stand out the index finger on it, to localize the point of maximum impulse and assess the extent of its thrust. It can be graded as just palpable, lifting, thrusting (stronger than lifting) or heaving.

- **Feel for any thrills:** Palpation with your hand on different areas will detect a tapping impulse, especially over the mitral and pulmonary area.

- **Parasternal heave:** Place the flat of your right palm parasternally over the right ventricular area and apply sustained and gentle pressure. If right ventricular hypertrophy is present, you will feel the heel of your hand lifted by its force.

Percussion is not necessary here.

Auscultation

1. **Mitral:** Ask patient to turn to the left side. Auscultate first with the diaphragm then with the bell.

2. **Tricuspid:** Use the diaphragm.

3. **Pulmonary:** Use the diaphragm. Listen for any splitting of sounds on deep inspiration.

4. **Aortic:** Use the diaphragm. Ask the patient to lean forward and hold their breath in deep expiration.

5. **Auscultate** the base of the lungs for crepitations.

Mention that you would like to complete the examination by taking the patient's blood pressure and examine for any hepatomegaly.

- Ask the patient to dress.

- Thank the patient and the examiner.

GASTROINTESTINAL

Task: Examine the gastrointestinal system of this 48-year-old man admitted to your ward.

Suggested approach

- Introduce yourself to the patient.

- Confirm the identity of the patient.

- Obtain verbal consent from the patient.

- Ensure privacy and achieve adequate exposure.

- In case of females, do not forget to ask for a chaperone.

- Ask patient to lower his trousers as often Pfannenstiel's incisions are missed.

General examination

- **Nails** – Pallor/clubbing/cyanosis/leuconychia

- **Palm** – Palmar erythema/Dupuytren's contracture/flapping tremors

- **Pulse** – Rate and rhythm

- **Eye** – Jaundice and pallor

- **Tongue** – Pallor, cyanosis and fetor hepaticus

- **Oedema** – Ankle, but mention that you would like to look for sacral oedema

- **Chest** – Gynaecomastia, loss of chest or axillary hair and spider naevi (check hands, arms, face, chest and back).

Systemic examination

Inspection

- Shape of the abdomen

- Type of respiration

- Position of umbilicus

- Swelling, redness, scars and sinuses in the abdomen

- Visible pulsations in the abdomen
- Caput medusa with other venous engorgement
- Abdominal swelling, abdominal distension (in one particular area)
- Distended abdominal veins.

Palpation

- Palpate abdomen for guarding, rigidity and tenderness.
- Palpate the neck and supraclavicular fossae for cervical lymph nodes.
- If you do not find lymph nodes then proceed to examine the axillae and groins for evidence of generalized lymphadenopathy.
- Feel for any obvious mass.

Palpate organs

Liver: Start in the right iliac fossa working upwards to the right hypochondrium. The liver is felt against the radial border of the index finger and the pulps of the index and middle fingers as they descend on inspiration, at which time you can gently press and move upwards to meet them.

Spleen: Start in the right iliac fossa moving diagonally across the abdomen to the left hypochondrium. The spleen is felt against the radial border of the index finger and the pulps of the index and middle fingers as they descend on inspiration, at which time you can gently press and move upwards to meet them.

Kidneys: It is done through bimanual palpation of each lateral region. Try to feel it by blotting a hand on back and front and push forward – if it is enlarged you can feel it butting the hand in front and it moves only slightly on inspiration.

Test for ascites – fluid thrill: A fluid thrill can be elicited when one side of the abdomen is tapped with one hand. A 'splash' can be detected on the other side of the abdomen by placing your other hand there.

Percussion

- **Liver and splenic dullness:** The percussion must be used from the nipple downwards on both sides to locate the upper edge of the liver on the right and spleen on the left.
- **Shifting dullness:** 'shifting' or 'moving' dullness – the fluid moves as the patient moves, and thus dullness shifts. Tap across the abdomen to see if there is an area of dullness that moves when the patient moves.

Auscultation

- For bowel sounds

- Aortic and renal bruit.

■ Conclude the examination by mentioning per rectal examination and hernial orifices.

■ Ask patient to dress and thank the patient and the examiner.

RESPIRATORY SYSTEM

Task: Examine the respiratory system of this 43-year-old man admitted to your ward.

Suggested approach

- Introduce yourself to the patient.
- Confirm the identity of the patient.
- Obtain verbal consent from the patient.
- Ensure privacy and achieve adequate exposure.
- In case of females, do not forget to ask for a chaperone.

General examination

- **Nails** – Pallor/clubbing/cyanosis
- **Pulse** – Rate, rhythm and volume
- **Eye** – Jaundice and pallor
- **Tongue** – Pallor and cyanosis.

Systemic examination

Inspection

1. Movement of the chest
2. Deformity
3. Respiratory rate
4. Respiratory pattern – abdominothoracic or reverse
5. Visible pulsations and apex beat
6. Accessory muscles of respiration – if accessory muscles are being used during breathing
7. Redness, scars, sinuses and engorged veins.

Palpation

Remember to ask permission before touching the patient.

a. Tracheal position

Inform the patient that you will be pressing on his airway and it will cause him some discomfort. Then place the index and ring fingers on the manubrium sternae over the prominent points on either side. Use the middle finger to gently feel the tracheal rings to detect either deviation or tracheal tug.

b. Respiratory movements to check

- Anterior part: Supramammary and inframammary region
- Posterior: Interscapular and subscapular region
- Lateral: axillary region.

Chest expansion: To assess chest expansion first in the inframammary and then in the supramammary regions. Note the distance between each thumb and the midline and between both thumbs and try to assess the expansion in centimetres. Check both the front and back portion of the chest.

Chest asymmetry: Rest one hand lightly on either side of the front of the chest to see if there is any diminution of movements. Next grip the chest symmetrically with the fingertips in the rib spaces on either side and approximate the thumbs to meet in the middle in a straight horizontal line to see if there is any diminution of movements. Check both the front and back portion of the chest.

c. Tactile vocal fremitus

This can be tested by placing the ulnar aspect of the hand applied to the chest. Ask the patient to say "99" while feeling with the ulnar side of the hand at 6 percussion points.

d. Palpate for localisation of apex beat

Percussion

- Tell patient that you will be tapping on his chest, but won't be hurting him. Tell him to feel free to say 'stop' if this is uncomfortable.
- Areas to be percussed – direct percussion over the clavicle then follow same areas of palpation. Do not forget the lateral aspect over the axilla and posterior aspect.

Auscultation

Ensure that the patient breathes with the mouth open, regularly and deeply.

- Same areas as for palpation and percussion. Check for vocal resonance in all the areas.

- Mention any adventitious sounds and basal crepitations.

- Conclude that you would ideally check for upper respiratory tract pathologies and cervical lymph nodes.

- Do not forget to ask the patient to dress and thank him and examiner.

ALCOHOL MISUSE – PHYSICAL EXAMINATION

Task: Mr Brown is a 45-year-old man who is a known alcoholic and was admitted earlier this morning because of his heavy alcohol misuse. He has not yet had a physical examination. Given his history, conduct an appropriate physical examination. Explain to the examiners what you are looking for.

Suggested approach

- Introduce yourself to the patient.
- Confirm the identity of the patient.
- Obtain verbal consent from the patient.
- Ensure privacy and achieve adequate exposure.
- In case of females, do not forget to ask for a chaperone.
- **Briefly ask for symptoms of alcohol withdrawal** like tremors, sweating, agitation, restlessness and feeling anxious.

Examine the patient from the end of the bed

Look for classical stigmata, such as:

- Jaundice
- Abdominal distension
- Spider naevi, mainly on trunk, face and arms
- Caput medusae (dilated veins on the abdominal wall)
- Gynaecomastia.

General examination

Skin

Abrasions, bruises, scars suggestive of falls or violence.

Hair

Decreased body hair.

Face

- Facial redness
- Bilateral parotid enlargement.

Eyes

- Icterus
- Pallor
- Check for nystagmus.

Hands

- Leuconychia
- Clubbing
- Palmar erythema
- Dupuytren's contracture
- Ask patient to bend both hands back, looking for asterixis (flapping tremor).

Systemic examination

Cardiovascular examination

- Check pulse for tachycardia
- Check blood pressure for evidence of hypertension (raised in heavy alcohol misuse)
- Precordial examination and auscultation
- Peripheral oedema (heart failure seen with heavy alcohol misuse).

Respiratory examination

- Respiratory rate – orthopnoea.

Abdominal examination

Check for:

- Asymmetry
- Ascites
- Palpable liver (hepatomegaly) and look for tenderness in the epigastric and right hypochondriac regions.
- Testicular atrophy (males).

Neurological examination

Motor examination

- **Bulk and tone:** Look for muscle wasting

- **Power:** Loss of power with heavy drinking; quadriplegia

- **Reflexes:** Increased deep tendon reflexes

- **Abnormal movements:** Tremor seen in acute alcohol withdrawal (delirium tremens) and and also check for myoclonus

- **Co-ordination and gait:** Ataxia (cerebellar damage, Wernicke's syndrome).

Sensory examination

- Sensation: Altered sensations and/or loss of pain sensation in the limbs and trunk.

Other cortical functions

- Speech – dysarthria

- Vision – loss of visual acuity (optic atrophy)

- Orientation – confusion seen in a variety of alcohol-induced states.

- **Do not forget to ask the patient to dress.**

- **Thank the patient and the examiner.**

OPIATE WITHDRAWAL – PHYSICAL EXAMINATION

Task: You are called to see a 29-year-old man with a long history of heroin abuse who presented to the hospital last night. Assess him for features of opiate withdrawal, explaining to the examiner what you are looking for.

Suggested approach

- Introduce yourself to the patient.
- Confirm the identity of the patient.
- Obtain verbal consent from the patient.
- Ensure privacy and achieve adequate exposure.
- In case of females, do not forget to ask for a chaperone.

Ask about the following symptoms: craving, arthralgia, myalgia, abdominal cramps, vomiting and diarrhoea.
Observe for signs of withdrawal:

- Agitation
- Anxiety/irritability
- Restlessness (observation during assessment)
- Sweating
- Tremor (observation of outstretched hands).

General examination

Skin

- Sweating
- Piloerection (gooseflesh skin, necessary to feel skin)
- Abrasions, bruises, scars suggestive of falls or violence
- Scratch marks.

Eyes

- Dilated pupils
- Watery eyes (lacrimation)
- Icterus.

Face

- Rhinorrhoea, not accounted for by cold symptoms or allergies (observation during assessment)
- Yawning (observation during assessment).

Examine for:

- Injection sites (elbow, thighs etc.)
- Scars, infection, ulcers, abscesses or other signs of local inflammation.

Others to be checked for:

- Fever (if thermometer is not available, candidate should ask)
- Hyperglycaemia – obtain consent to do random blood glucose testing (hyperglycaemia in withdrawals – at least worth mentioning in the examination).

Systemic examination

Cardiovascular examination

- Check blood pressure for hyper/hypotension
- Check the pulse rate for tachycardia
- Auscultation for murmurs.

Respiratory system examination

- Respiratory rate: tachypnoea
- Any signs of infection in the respiratory tract.

Abdominal examination

- Hepatomegaly
- Splenomegaly.

Neurological examination

- Muscle tone and power – look for muscle wasting
- Reflexes
- Gait and co-ordination
- Peripheral sensation.

- Do not forget to ask patient to dress.
- Thank the patient and the examiner.

EATING DISORDER – PHYSICAL EXAMINATION

Task: Miss Pang is an 18-year-old woman who was admitted earlier today because of problems with eating and weight loss. Given her history, please conduct an appropriate physical examination. Explain to the examiners what you are looking for.

Suggested approach

- Introduce yourself to the patient.
- Confirm the identity of the patient.
- Obtain verbal consent from the patient.
- Ensure privacy and achieve adequate exposure.
- In case of females, do not forget to ask for a chaperone.
- Measure the patient's weight (if scales are available).
- Measure the patient's height (if equipment is available).

General examination

Skin

- Purpuric rash
- Signs of dehydration, areas of skin breakdown
- Skin tone – possibility of hypercarotinaemia
- Any signs of infection.

Hands and arms

- Palmar creases for pallor
- Brittle hair and nails.

Hair

- Look for lanugo hair (may be seen on arms, but typically on trunk)
- Normal secondary sexual hair pattern is unaffected.

Eyes

Look for pallor.

Cardiovascular examination

- Check pulse for bradycardia
- Check blood pressure for hypotension
- Carry out precordial examination and auscultation
- Look for peripheral oedema (may be seen).

Respiratory examination

Gastrointestinal examination

- Look in mouth for:
  a. Signs of dehydration
  b. Dental caries
  c. Damaged enamel from vomiting
  d. Incisor damage from self-induced vomiting with fingers
  e. Swollen salivary glands.
- Abdominal distension (constipation, acute gastric dilatation)
- Tenderness over the abdominal area (acute pancreatitis).

Neurological examination

Check for altered sensations (peripheral neuropathy).

Other test

'Squat test' – ability of patient to rise from squatting position unaided.

- Do not forget to ask the patient to dress.

- Thank the patient and the examiner.

ECT – ELECTRODE PLACEMENT

Task: You are requested to administer ECT to Mr X, who has consented to the procedure. Proceed to administer ECT to the mannequin, explaining the steps you take to the examiner. Assume that the appropriate dose has been set up and indicate the electrode placement for unilateral and bilateral ECT administration. Using the strip of EEG provided, indicate the different phases of the seizure.

What is expected?

- Knowledge of ECT administration procedures
- Correct electrode placement
- EEG interpretation.

There is no need to speak to the mannequin, but you are expected to run through the steps with the examiner.

Suggested approach

- Greet the patient and introduce yourself.
- Obtain permission before you proceed.
- Check that it is the correct 'patient' and confirm the identity of the patient.
- Check documentation to see that the patient has consented and **ECT consent form** has been duly signed, or if on a section of the Mental Health Act, appropriate forms have been filled out.
- Ask for consent again and briefly explain the procedure.
- Check that the pre-ECT form has been filled in, with emphasis on **nil by mouth** for at least 6 hours prior to ECT.
- Check that the **physical examination** has been done prior to ECT, all necessary **investigations** duly completed and anaesthetic opinion obtained.
- Check the **medical notes** to ensure that the psychiatric team has seen him after the last treatment to record progress and any adverse effects of ECT (if any after the last treatment).
- Check the **treatment card** to check for current medications.
- Make sure that the **appropriate dose has been set up** and once the patient is anaesthetized the ECT electrodes should be placed accordingly and the treatment is administered.
- Indicate the electrode placement for unilateral and bilateral ECT (see below).

- During treatment, also observe the nature, type and duration of the seizures.

- Make sure that you have documented the current used, type and duration of seizures, and any complications that arose, in the medical notes and on the ECT form.

- Make sure that the patient is taken to the recovery room accompanied by a nurse and the vital signs are being monitored.

- Comment on your findings to the examiner as well as the EEG interpretation.

- Thank the examiner at the end and leave the station.

Electrode positions

Bilateral: 4 cm above the midpoint of the line between the external auditory meatus and the lateral angle of the eye.

Unilateral: The first electrode is placed on the nondominant side, 4 cm above the midpoint of the line between external angle of the eye and the external auditory meatus. The second electrode is placed 10 cm above the first, vertically above the meatus on the same side.

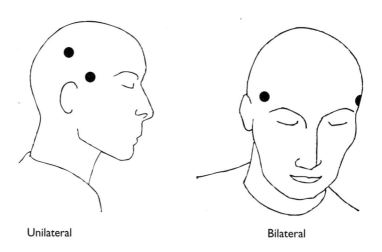

Unilateral   Bilateral

EEG interpretation

Look for the stimulus on the EEG record. The EEG usually develops patterned sequences consisting of high voltage sharp waves and spikes, followed by rhythmic slow waves that end abruptly in a well-defined endpoint.

ECG RECORDING

Task: You have been asked to perform a routine ECG on this 'patient'. Explain the procedure as you would to a real patient and place the ECG electrodes on the mannequin. Provide a brief report to the examiner on the ECG trace provided.

What is expected?

- Knowledge of placement of the ECG leads

- Information to be given to the patient about the procedure

- Reporting an ECG trace.

Suggested approach

- Greet the 'patient' and introduce yourself.

- Explain briefly what you are going to do and take consent, for example, 'Mr G, I have been asked to do a routine ECG for you. This involves me placing some electrodes on your chest, arms and legs. I'll be connecting these leads to a machine, which will record the electrical activity of your heart, which is the ECG trace. This is a painless, non-invasive procedure taking about 5 minutes.'

- Reassure him that this procedure does not involve passing electric current through him, and the procedure itself causes minimal discomfort.

- 'I hope you have no objections to my recording your ECG.'

- Reassure the 'patient' that the procedure will be stopped if he or she is uncomfortable at any stage.

Positions of limb leads and chest leads

Standard chest lead positions
- V1 – Fourth intercostal space, right sternal edge

- V2 – Fourth intercostal space, left sternal edge

- V3 – Half way between the second and fourth electrodes

- V4 – Fifth intercostal space in the mid-clavicular line

- V5 – Fifth intercostal space in the anterior axillary line

- V6 – In line with V5 in the midaxillary line.

Limb lead positions

- One on each arm, on the palmar aspect of the wrists
- One on either ankle, on the medial side.
  1. Attach the limb leads to all four limbs, using contact gel under each electrode.
  2. Ensure good contact with the skin.
  3. Switch on the machine and make the recording. Once completed, dispose of the electrode pads and waste appropriately.

Usually a mannequin with clear bony markings is provided, so it requires a correct identification of the intercostal space.

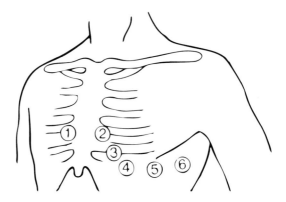

■ Thank the 'patient' for his co-operation.

INTERPRETATION OF ECG

Task: Comment on the routine ECG tracing of a 50-year-old person with a history of paranoid schizophrenia being treated with an antipsychotic drug. Comment on the ECG. √

Comment on the following:

- Rate
- Rhythm
- Regularity
- Axis
- P wave
- PR interval
- QRS complex
- Q waves
- ST segment
- T wave
- QT interval
- Abnormalities
- Opinion
- Management plan.

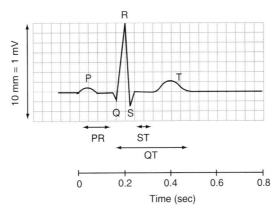

P wave (0.08–0.10 s)   QRS (0.06–0.10 s)

P–R interval (0.12–0.20 s)   Q–T$_c$ interval (≤0.44 s)*

$$*QT_c = \frac{QT}{\sqrt{RR}}$$

Comment on the following:

Rate

Divide 300 by the number of large squares between each QRS complex (or) between two RR intervals.

Rhythm

If a P wave is seen, then it is a sinus rhythm. Otherwise it is a non-sinus rhythm.

Regularity

This can be regular or irregular. To assess rhythm, lay a card along an ECG and mark the position of three successive R waves. Slide the card back and forth to check that all the intervals are the same.

Axis

- The normal axis lies between −30 degrees and +90 degrees.
- If the QRS complexes in leads I and II are predominantly positive, the axis is normal.
- Left axis deviation exists if lead I is positive, and both leads II and aVF are negative.
- Right axis deviation occurs if lead I is negative, and leads II and aVF are positive.

P wave

This is caused by depolarisation of the atria. Normal height and width are less than 2.5 mm, and 0.11 s, respectively, in lead II. Comment on whether it is too wide, or too tall.

PR interval

The range is 0.12–0.20 s, or 3–5 small squares. This should be less than 5 small squares, or else it is prolonged.

QRS complex

The QRS complex represents ventricular depolarisation. Its duration is less than 0.12 s, or less than 3 small squares. If more than 0.12 s, a conduction defect is likely.

Q waves

These are pathological if they are more than 25% of the height of the following R wave, and more than 0.04 s wide (1 small square).

ST segment

This is normally isoelectric (flat). It can become elevated acutely in myocardial infarction or pericarditis. ST depression occurs in several conditions including myocardial ischaemia and left ventricular hypertrophy.

ST elevation is significant if there are >1 mm elevation in limb leads and >2 mm elevation in chest leads.

T wave

The T wave represents ventricular repolarisation. T wave inversion in leads I, II, or V 4–6 is usually abnormal. Peaked T waves can occur in hyperkalemia. T wave can be flattened in hypokalemia.

QT interval

This is the interval between the beginning of the QRS complex and the end of the T wave. It varies with heart rate, and so must be corrected – the QT_c, or corrected QT interval.

To calculate the QT_c, divide the QT interval by the square root of the preceding R-R interval (the latter is the interval between the R waves of two successive QRS complexes). It should be less than 0.42 seconds.

- Corrected QT_c = QT/square root of R-R interval in seconds.

- Corrected QT_c should be approximately 2 large squares.

ECG interpretation

The abnormalities would usually be very evident, so think of common things. If you can't make out any specific abnormality, then report the findings as above and then mention whether you think the ECG is normal or abnormal.

CARDIOPULMONARY RESUSCITATION (CPR)

Task: Perform CPR on this collapsed patient on your ward. Usually the task comes as: 'Please provide BLS to this patient who has been found collapsed in the ward (or on the road)'.

This is a strictly dummy station and here there is no need to identify the patient or introduce yourself to the patient.

Follow the steps in strict order

1. Is it safe to approach? Is there any trauma?

2. After assuming that there is no trauma and the patient is safe, go near the mannequin. Shake him by his shoulders and ask loudly at the same time: 'Hello, hello, can you hear me?' or 'Are you OK?'

3. If there is no response, shout for help – 'Help, Help!' Often the dummies in this station are clad with jumpers or other clothes, so remember to undress the dummy above the waist.

4. Check for a **patent airway** to rule out any foreign body, secretions, etc. If the airways are clear, tilt the head, lift the chin.

5. Keeping the airways open, look, listen and feel for normal breathing.

   - Look for chest movement

   - Listen at the victim's mouth for breath sounds

   - Feel for air on your cheek

     Look, listen and feel for no more than 10 secs to determine if the victim is breathing normally.

6. If he is not breathing normally, activate the emergency alarm system and dial '999'. Start 'chest compression' as follows:

   Kneel by the side of the victim, place the heel of one hand in the centre of the victim's chest, and place the heel of your other hand on top of the first hand. Interlock the fingers of your hands, position yourself vertically above the victim's chest and, with arms straight, press down on the sternum 4–5 cm. Following each compression, release all the pressure on the chest without losing contact between your hands and the sternum.

7. After 30 compressions, open the airway again using head tilt and chin lift.

8. Now give two effective 'rescue breaths'. Maintain the head tilt, chin lift position, then pinch the nose and purse your lips tightly on the mannequin's lips. Blow as forcefully as possible watching for chest expansion.

9. Then return your hands, without delay, to the correct position on the sternum and give a further 30 chest compressions.

10. Continue with chest compressions and rescue breaths in a ratio of 30:2.

11. Stop to recheck the victim only if he starts breathing normally. Otherwise, do not interrupt resuscitation.

12. Repeat the same cycle (**30 chest compressions: 2 breaths**) until:

    a. The patient responds

    b. Help arrives, or

    c. You are exhausted.

13. Once the patient is responsive, put him in the left lateral position, i.e. the **recovery position**.

    A little modification is needed for some special situations such as:

    ● In cases of trauma, we do not tilt the head in case the cervical spine is injured. Instead we give a jaw thrust to open the airway.

    ● With children, in cases of drowning and primary respiratory failure, continue rescue breaths for 1 minute and if still unresponsive, then activate the alarm system. This is because in all of the above if respiratory arrest is reversed, the patient will not need cardiac resuscitation.

FUNDOSCOPY

Task: Perform an ophthalmoscopic examination on this 49-year-old man and describe your findings and interpretation to the examiner.

What is expected?

- Clear instructions prior to performing an ophthalmoscopic examination
- Appropriate use of ophthalmoscope
- Findings
- Diagnosis.

Suggested approach

- Greet the patient and introduce yourself.
- Confirm if you have to address the examiner or the patient.
- Explain the purpose of the visit.
- Obtain permission before you proceed.

Explain that:

- You have to look into the back of the patient's eyes using this light.
- You have to do it with the light in the room switched off.
- The light can be uncomfortable.
- You will have to come so close to the patient that your face may touch his. Get the patient's permission.
- Ensure that the ophthalmoscope is working. Turn it on. Check the light.
- Ask the patient to remove his glasses and look at an object at a distance and at eye level, and to blink and breathe normally.
- Either keep your own glasses/lenses or remove your glasses/lenses and dial up the appropriate lens for your refractive error; – lenses for myopia and + lenses for hypermetropia.
- Stand or sit on the side to be examined at 1 metre from the patient and with eyes level with the patient's. Ask the patient to stare at a fixed point in the distance.
- With the right hand holding the ophthalmoscope, approach the patient's right side at an angle of about 15 degrees, nasally and inwards and at a

distance of 30 cm. Ensure that you use your right eye to examine the patient's right eye and your left eye to examine the patient's left eye.

- Consider your eye and the ophthalmoscope functioning as a single unit. Bring your eye slowly towards the patient's eye until you are as close as possible without touching the eyelashes.

- The back of the patient's eye should be in focus.

- Look systematically – start with the lens, then vitreous, followed by the disc, vessels in the centre, in each quadrant and then the macula.

- When the retina is in focus, follow a blood vessel to the optic disc. The optic disc is slightly pink with sharp borders and a central cup. Look at the four arteries and the accompanying veins, especially where they cross each other. Look for pallor, swelling, new vessel formation, exudates and haemorrhages.

- Locate any abnormality as though the fundus is a clock with the disc at the centre. The diameter of the disc (1.5 mm) is used as the unit of measurement. For example, hard exudates at 4, 6 and 9 o'clock, 2–3 disc diameters from the disc.

- Look at the macula by asking the patient to look directly at the light and using a narrow beam.

Examine both eyes.

The findings should be given in the same order as the examination. Even if the diagnosis is obvious, first inform the findings first, and then give the diagnosis.

■ Thank the patient and the examiner.

The common slides that are usually kept in the examinations are:

1. Normal fundus

2. Papilloedema

3. Diabetic retinopathy

4. Hypertensive retinopathy.

Interpretation of Blood Results and Management

NEUROLEPTIC MALIGNANT SYNDROME

Task: You are asked to see a 29-year-old man who has become increasingly physically unwell over the last 48 hours. He is sweaty, agitated, and a little tremulous.

Current medication

1. Zuclopenthixol decanoate 300 mg weekly. He was started on this medication 2 weeks previously.

2. Procyclidine 5 mg bid.

Blood results

FBC 15.8; WCC 17.8; platelets 387; Na 144; Cl 103; K 3.9; urea 8.3; creatinine 102.

Vital signs

Temperature 38.2°C, BP 144/100, HR 109/min.

In this station, you may be asked to discuss the possible diagnosis, investigations and management with a senior colleague or consultant.

Questions

1. What is the most likely diagnosis?

2. What are the other symptoms and signs of this condition?

3. What are the risk factors causing this condition?

4. What other investigations would you like to do?

5. How would you manage this condition?

6. What about prescribing antipsychotics in the future?

7. When do you prefer ECT treatment for neuroleptic malignant syndrome (NMS)?

Answers

1. Possible neuroleptic malignant syndrome

2. Signs and symptoms

- Symptoms: Fever, diaphoresis, rigidity, confusion, fluctuating consciousness, fluctuating blood pressure, tachycardia

- Signs: Elevated creatinine kinase, leucocytosis, and altered liver function tests.

3. Risk factors

- High potency typical antipsychotic drugs
- Recent or rapid dose increase of antipsychotics
- Rapid dose reduction
- Abrupt withdrawal of anticholinergic drugs
- Psychosis, organic brain disease, alcoholism, Parkinson's disease
- Hyperthyroidism
- Agitation
- Dehydration.

4. Investigations

- Blood tests include:

    a. Creatinine phosphokinase (CK) – elevated

    b. Arterial blood gases (looking for metabolic acidosis)

    c. Coagulation screen

    d. Serum iron (has been reported to be low).

- EEG: Non-focal generalized slowing on electroencephalography, consistent with encephalopathy, has been reported in over half of NMS cases

- CT scan

- Lumbar puncture.

Cerebrospinal fluid examinations, sepsis evaluation, and brain-imaging studies are negative in NMS, and allow for the exclusion of other causes of fever and neurological deterioration.

5. Management

In the psychiatric unit:

a. Withdraw antipsychotics (offending drug)

b. Monitor temperature, pulse, BP

c. Possible transfer to the medical unit if patient shows evidence of further deterioration in his/her physical health status.

In the medical unit:

- Rehydration
- Sedation with **benzodiazepines**, which are useful in reversing catatonia, are easy to administer, and can be tried initially in most cases
- Trials of **bromocriptine, amantadine,** or other dopamine agonists may be tried in patients with moderate symptoms of NMS
- **Dantrolene sodium** appears to be beneficial in cases of NMS involving significant rigidity and hyperthermia. It has been beneficial in rapidly reducing extreme temperature elevations in many cases
- **Artificial ventilation** if required
- **L-dopa** and **carbamazepine** have also been used
- Consider **ECT** for treatment after other interventions have failed.

6. Restarting

- Antipsychotic treatment will be required in most instances and 'antipsychotics rechallenge' is associated with acceptable risk
- Stop antipsychotics for at least 5–7 days, preferably longer
- Allow time for symptoms and signs to resolve completely
- Begin with very small dose and increase very slowly with close monitoring of temperature, pulse and blood pressure
- CK monitoring may be useful
- Consider using an antipsychotic structurally unrelated to that associated with NMS or a drug with low dopamine affinity (quetiapine or clozapine)
- Avoid depots and high potency conventional antipsychotics for the future.

7. ECT may be preferred

a. If NMS symptoms are refractory to other measures

b. In patients with prominent catatonic features

c. In patients who develop a residual catatonic state or remain psychotic after NMS has resolved.

SEROTONIN SYNDROME

Task: Whilst on call, you are asked to see a 32-year-old man who has been becoming more physically unwell over the last 24 hours. He is not your patient, but you know that his antidepressants have very recently been changed. His symptoms are confusion, restlessness, agitation, sweating and shivering.

Questions

1. What is the most likely diagnosis?

2. What other information would you like?

3. What other findings would you look for?

4. How would you manage him?

In this station, you may be asked to discuss the possible diagnosis and management with a senior colleague or consultant.

Answers

1. Serotonin syndrome

2. Important information would include:

a. Previous antidepressants, their dose, and duration of treatment, possible side effects and response to medication

b. New antidepressants, their dose, and duration of treatment

c. Length of 'washout' period, if any

d. Previous reactions or intolerance to medications.

3. Other findings to look for would include:

a. Fever

b. Tachycardia

c. Myoclonus

d. Hyperreflexia

e. Incoordination

f. Oculogyric crisis (rare).

4. Treatment involves:

a. Monitoring of physical condition

b. Stopping any serotonergic drugs, especially antidepressants

c. Discussion with medical colleagues and transfer if condition deteriorates

d. Treatment steps in the medical unit may involve:

- Close monitoring of vital signs.
- Proper hydration, i.v. fluids (if necessary)
- Cooling blankets for hyperthermia
- Anticonvulsants for seizures
- Intramuscular chlorpromazine as an antipyretic and sedative agent
- Clonazepam for myoclonus
- Nifedipine for hypertension
- Artificial ventilation for respiratory insufficiency.

EATING DISORDER

Task: A 19-year-old girl is seen at the outpatient clinic. She presented with severe weight loss and abnormal eating patterns. Her weight was 30 kg and her height was 175 cm.

Physical findings

Pulse 56 bpm
BP 86/62 mmHg
Temperature 36.2°C

Her blood results include the following:

Haematology		Biochemistry	
Hb	9.3	Sodium	129
WC	3.5	Potassium	3.2
Platelets	137	Chloride	97
MCV	94.3	Urea	8.5
MCH	Not available	Creatinine	138
Haematocrit	0.28	Calcium	2.01
ESR	2	Magnesium	0.65
		Phosphate	0.63
		Glucose random	3.4
		Creatinine kinase	187

Liver function tests		Thyroid function tests	
AST	47	TSH	0.03
ALT	58	T_4	25.7
Alk phos	135	T_3	Not available
Bilirubin	25		
GGT	64		
Albumin	35		

In this station, you may be asked to discuss the possible diagnosis; investigations and management plan with a senior colleague or consultant.

Questions

1. Looking at the list of investigations, identify if there are any abnormalities and what do you think is the likely diagnosis?

2. What investigations would you do routinely in a patient with anorexia nervosa?

3. What are the endocrine changes that can be expected in a patient with anorexia nervosa?

4. What are the metabolic abnormalities and blood changes that can be expected in a patient with anorexia nervosa?

5. What are the cardiac and gastrointestinal complications that can be expected in a patient with anorexia nervosa?

6. What other abnormalities might you expect to find?

7. When would you consider inpatient treatment?

8. What would be your management plan for this patient with anorexia nervosa?

9. What kinds of psychological interventions would be helpful?

Suggested answers

1. The abnormalities identified include:

- Low body mass index
- Bradycardia
- Hypotension
- Anaemia
- Leucopenia
- Thrombocytopenia
- Hyponatraemia
- Hypokalemia
- Low calcium, phosphate, and magnesium
- Abnormal LFTs
- High T_4 with suppressed TSH.

The most probable diagnosis is **anorexia nervosa**.

2. Essential investigations would comprise:

a. FBC

b. U&E

c. Glucose

d. LFTs

e. TFTs

f. Vitamin B and folate levels

g. Serum calcium, magnesium, phosphate

h. ECG.

3. Possible endocrine changes that can be expected are:

- Raised growth hormone level
- Cortisol (positive DST) level raised
- Gonadotrophin levels decreased
- Oestrogen level decreased
- Testosterone level decreased
- T_3 (sick euthyroid syndrome) levels decreased
- Amenorrhoea/loss of libido.

4. Metabolic abnormalities that can be expected are:

- Dehydration
- Hypoglycaemia (due to bingeing and purging) and impaired glucose tolerance (due to starvation)
- Hypercholesterolemia
- Hypokalemia
- Hypoproteinemia
- Deranged LFTs
- Plasma amylase (raised)
- Lowered calcium, magnesium and phosphate levels
- Hypothermia.

Haematological:

- Normochromic, normocytic, or iron-deficient anaemia
- Leucopenia, with a relative lymphocytosis
- Thrombocytopenia
- Low ESR
- Hypocellular marrow
- Reduced serum complement level.

5. Cardiovascular and gastrointestinal complications include:

Cardiovascular:

- Bradycardia
- Hypotension
- Peripheral oedema
- Congestive cardiac failure
- Decreased heart size
- QT prolongation.

Gastrointestinal:

- Swollen salivary glands
- Dental caries
- Erosion of enamel (as a result of vomiting)
- Delayed gastric emptying
- Acute gastric dilations (bulimic episodes, vigorous refeeding, constipation)
- Acute pancreatitis.

6. Other complications of anorexia include:

Neurological:

- EEG abnormalities
- Seizures
- Peripheral neuropathy
- Cerebral oedema.

Renal:

- Proteinuria
- Reduced GFR
- Acute/chronic renal failure
- Hypokalemic nephropathy.

Musculoskeletal:

- Stunted growth
- Muscle cramps

- Proximal myopathy
- Osteoporosis
- Pathological fractures.

7. Inpatient treatment will be considered if:

Article I

a. BMI less than 13.5

b. Severe suicidal risk and severe depression

c. Rapid weight loss with the patient's weight dangerously low

d. Electrolyte imbalance leading to ECG changes (low potassium <3 mmol/L)

e. Crisis situation

f. Failed out patient care (non-compliance).

8. General management

Medical

- I would consider treating her as an inpatient and I would offer informal admission but if the patient refuses then I would consider compulsory treatment under mental health legislation.

- Hospitalize the patient for weight restoration and monitor as part of the medical management. It is reasonable to aim for a weight gain of between 0.5 and 1 kg each week, and weight restoration takes between 8 and 12 weeks.

- Rehydration and correction of serum electrolytes.

- Instigate nutritional rehabilitation and involve the dietician for nutritional counselling: Aim for a target weight, refeeding programme – a balanced diet of 2500–3000 kcal/day provided as three or four meals a day with supplementary snacks.

Nursing

- Offer support at meal times; monitor her food intake.

- The eating pattern should be supervized by a nurse to provide support and reassurance. Ensure that the patient does not induce vomiting (or) take purgatives.

- Monitor for suicidality and impulsive behaviour.

9. Psychological interventions

Educating the patient and their family about the disorder and its treatment is important, including health hazards of weight loss and starvation.

Behaviour programme – focuses on positive reinforcement and encouragement of positive behaviour.

CBT: The psychologist would attempt cognitive restructuring to identify automatic negative thoughts and to challenge core beliefs. CBT has been particularly used with the aim of modifying abnormal cognitions about shape, weight and eating and the behavioural component focuses on behavioural experiments including self-monitoring of weight, goal setting, assertiveness training and relaxation.

Family therapy and parental counselling – to look for factors like overprotectiveness, enmeshment and lack of conflict resolution and provide more family support if necessary.

Miscellaneous Topics

RAPID TRANQUILLIZATION

Task: Mr Jason Deal is a 28-year-old man admitted to the acute psychiatric ward in a very disturbed state. He was agitated, restless, distressed, complained of hearing voices instructing to kill him or others. He shouted at the ward staff and other patients and remained quite intimidating.

You are the psychiatric doctor on call and they bleeped you to come and assess the patient. The staff members are concerned about him and want medication to be prescribed to calm him down. How will you manage the situation?

Acutely disturbed or violent behaviour

Management of an acutely disturbed or violent patient is one of the common clinical scenarios that we face in psychiatric wards, so this can be asked as a separate station.

Acute behavioural disturbance can occur in the context of psychiatric illness, physical illness, substance abuse or personality disorder. Psychotic symptoms are common and the patient may be aggressive towards others, secondary to persecutory delusions or auditory, visual or tactile hallucinations.

Plans for the management of individual patients should ideally be made in advance. The aim is to prevent disturbed behaviour and reduce risk of violence.

Nursing interventions (de-escalation, time out), increased nursing levels, transfer of the patient to a psychiatric intensive care unit (PICU) or pharmacological management are all options that may be employed.

In the examination, the steps for rapid tranquillization (RT) can be asked as a series of questions by the consultant (steps 1–5, possible complications and remedial measures).

In an emergency situation:

Step 1

- De-escalation, time out, placement, etc., as appropriate.

Step 2

Offer oral treatment:

- Haloperidol 5 mg with or without lorazepam 1–2 mg (or)
- Olanzapine 10 mg with or without lorazepam 1–2 mg (or)
- Risperidone 1–2 mg with or without lorazepam 1–2 mg.

Repeat every 45–60 minutes. Go to step 3 if three doses fail.

Step 3

Consider consultation with senior colleague. Consider i.m. treatment. From this point onwards, review the patient's legal status. The requirement for enforced i.m. medication in informal patients should prompt the use of the Mental Health Act.

However in case of psychiatric emergencies, we can still treat patients under common law.

- Haloperidol 5 mg with or without lorazepam 1–2 mg (olanzapine 5–10 mg i.m. can also be used instead of haloperidol)

- Have flumazenil available to reverse the effects of lorazepam. (Monitor respiratory rate – give flumazenil if rate falls below 10/min.)

- Repeat i.m. haloperidol up to 3 times at 30-minute intervals, if insufficient effect.

Note: Promethazine 50 mg i.m. is an alternative in benzodiazepine-tolerant patients. Promethazine has a slow onset of action but is often an effective sedative. Dilution is not required before i.m. injection. May be repeated up to a maximum 100 mg/day. Wait 1–2 hours after injection to assess response.

Step 4

Consider consultation with a senior colleague. Consider i.v. treatment.

- Diazepam 10 mg over at least 5 minutes

- Repeat after 5–10 minutes if the effect is insufficient (up to three times).

Use diazemuls to avoid injection site reactions. I.v. therapy may be used instead of i.m. when a very rapid effect is required. I.v. therapy also ensures near immediate delivery of the drug to its site of action and effectively avoids the danger of inadvertent accumulation of slowly absorbed i.m. doses. Note also that i.v. doses can be repeated after only 5–10 minutes if no effect is observed.

Have flumazenil available to reverse the effects of diazepam. (Monitor respiratory rate – give flumazenil if the rate falls below 10/minute.)

Step 5

Seek expert advice.

- Amylobarbitone 250 mg i.m. or paraldehydes 5–10 ml i.m. are options.

Amylobarbitone is a powerful respiratory depressant with no pharmacological antagonist. Have facilities for mechanical ventilation available. Paraldehyde is now used extremely rarely and is difficult to obtain. It should be used when all else has failed.

In many cases, ECT may be more appropriate. Very few episodes of RT should reach this point.

Questions

What are the aims of rapid tranquillization?

The aims of rapid tranquillization are threefold:

1. To reduce suffering for the patient: psychological or physical (through self-harm or accidents)

2. To reduce risk of harm to others by maintaining a safe environment

3. To do no harm (by prescribing safe regimes and monitoring physical health).

How will you monitor a patient after parenteral drug administration?

After any parenteral drug administration monitor as follows:

- Temperature
- Pulse
- Blood pressure
- Respiratory rate.

Monitor every 5–10 minutes for 1 hour, then half-hourly until the patient is ambulatory.

Remedial measures in rapid tranquillization

Problem 1: Acute dystonia (including oculogyric crises)

- Remedial measures:

Give procyclidine 5–10 mg i.m. or i.v., or benzatropine 1–2 mg i.m.

Problem 2: Reduced respiratory rate (less than 10/minute) or oxygen saturation less than 90%

- Remedial measures:
  a. Give oxygen
  b. Raise legs
  c. Ensure the patient is not lying facing down

d. Give flumazenil, if benzodiazepine-induced respiratory depression is suspected

e. If induced by any other sedative agent, ventilate mechanically.

Problem 3: Irregular or slow pulse (less than 50 bpm)

● **Remedial measures:**
Refer to specialist medical care immediately.

Problem 4: Fall in blood pressure (>30 mmHg orthostatic drop or <50 mmHg diastolic)

● **Remedial measures:**

a. Lie patient flat, tilt bed towards head

b. Monitor closely.

Problem 5: Increased temperature

● **Remedial measures:**

a. Withhold antipsychotics: (risk of NMS and perhaps arrhythmias)

b. Check creatinine kinase urgently.

Other useful points

1. Choice depends on current treatment. If the patient is already on established antipsychotics, lorazepam may be used alone. If the patient uses street drugs or is already receiving benzodiazepines regularly, an antipsychotic may be used alone. For the majority of patients, the best response will be obtained with a combination of an antipsychotic and lorazepam.

2. Ensure that potential anticholinergics are available. Procyclidine 5–10 mg i.m. or benzatropine 1–2 mg i.m. may be required to reverse acute dystonic reactions.

3. Proceed with caution with the very young and elderly and those with pre-existing brain damage or impulse control problems as disinhibition reactions are more likely.

4. If the patient is asleep or unconscious, the use of pulse oximetry to continuously measure oxygen saturation is desirable.

5. A nurse should remain with the patient until they are ambulatory again.

6. ECG and haematological monitoring are also strongly recommended when parenteral antipsychotics are given, especially when higher doses are used.

TELEPHONE ADVICE ABOUT A CONFUSED PATIENT

Task: You are the psychiatric doctor on call and the surgical on-call doctor contacts you. He contacted you regarding a 52-year-old man who fractured his leg the day before and underwent major orthopaedic surgery.

Today, however, the patient has become very confused, restless, sweaty, and shaky and appeared to be very anxious. The surgical on-call doctor gave a history that the patient is a chronic alcoholic and has been drinking up to three bottles of whisky a day. He seems to have had no alcohol since admission. The surgical on-call doctor is concerned and has contacted you for further advice over the phone.

A. Introduce yourself to your colleague

B. Explore more history, which includes:

- Circumstances of the injury and admission

- Past psychiatric history and medications

- Medical history and medications

- Drug and alcohol history

- Current social situation.

C. Give priority to alcohol history

- Current usage and longitudinal history.

- Enquire for features of dependence syndrome.

- Enquire about withdrawal symptoms – both physical and psychological symptoms.

- Ask for symptoms of delirium tremens, which include clouding of consciousness, disorientation in time and place, poor attention span, visual hallucinations and illusions, which are often vivid and frightening. Tactile hallucinations of insects crawling over the body may occur.

- Ask for any autonomic disturbance, which includes fever, sweating, tachycardia, hypertension, and pupillary dilatation.

- Ask about neurological signs and symptoms.

245

D. Ask about their current management plan and what their team feels about the patient

Ask for necessary blood investigations and other investigations to rule out acute confusional state (FBC, ESR, blood culture, LFT, U&E, creatinine, TFT, chest X-ray, ECG, and urine C&S).

E. Give further management advice that includes:

- Treat the underling cause if any, such as infection, dehydration etc.

- Ensure adequate fluid and electrolyte balance, providing adequate nutrition

- Optimisation of environment – well-lit quiet room with adequate lighting

- Nursing support – consistent nursing support to offer reassurance, reorientation and explanation. If possible, discuss providing input from the psychiatric nursing team

- Librium sliding scale (detoxification regime with chlordiazepoxide (Librium) in a reducing dose)

- Using parenteral benzodiazepines to achieve quick sedation

- Instituting parenteral, high potency vitamins (thiamine supplementation or multivitamins)

- Avoiding use of phenothiazine antipsychotics (haloperidol) due to risk of inducing seizures

- Warn about the risk of withdrawal seizures and Wernicke's encephalopathy

- Offer to see patient if necessary.

ASSESS CAPACITY

Task: Mr White is a schoolteacher admitted to a general surgical ward in your hospital for acute abdominal pain. He had an ultrasound scan for abdominal pain. The scan picked up an appendicular mass, probably appendicular abscess. The surgeons have confirmed that there is a high risk of rupture of the abscess and suggested surgical removal of the abscess.

After the routine work-up and investigations, he has declined to go ahead with the operation, and he wishes to leave the hospital. The surgeons have asked you for advice as to whether he can go, given he has already signed the consent form.

The patient is worried that you will section him so that they can proceed with the operation. Assess his capacity/competency to refuse treatment and address his concern about being sectioned.

Mental Capacity Act

The Act defines capacity as follows:

An adult can be considered unable to make a particular decision if:

- He or she has an impairment of or disturbance in the functioning of the mind or brain, whether temporary or permanent.

and

He or she is unable to undertake any of the following steps:

- Understand the information relevant to the decision

- Retain that information

- Use or weigh that information as part of the decision-making process

- Communicate that decision made (by talking, sign language or other means).

Explore the following:

- The nature of the problem and proposed treatment

- Why someone has said that he/she needs it

- The treatment's principle risks and benefits

- The patient's ability to retain this information and make a reasoned decision

- The consequences of not receiving the proposed treatment

- Whether he or she has an impairment or disturbance in the functioning of the mind or brain
- Patient's reasons for refusing treatment (in this scenario).

Suggested approach

- Greet the patient and introduce yourself
- Explain the purpose of the visit
- Obtain permission before you proceed
- Address his/her main concerns
- Start with open questions
- Do not take a history.

Nature of problem and proposed treatment

- 'Tell me what you understand about the nature of the problem in your tummy?'
- 'Tell me what you understand about the treatment that has been planned?'

Why has someone said that he needs it?

- 'Why do you think that you need an operation?'
- 'Why do the surgeons think that you need an operation?'

Principle risks and benefits of treatment and consequences of not receiving the proposed treatment

Patient's understanding of the risks of the procedure

- 'Have you been told about the risks of having the operation?'
- 'Do you think that it might be painful/you may die?'

Patient's understanding of the risks of not having the procedure

- 'What do you think will happen to this swelling in the future?'
- 'Do you think that you will get better if nothing is done?'
- 'Can you tell me the pros and cons of the operation?'

Note: If the patient does not understand the relevant information then clarify it with the patient, address his queries, offer a clear explanation and give the information in simple, clear terms and then assess whether he has understood it.

Does the patient believe the above information?

1. 'Do you believe there is a problem in your tummy?'

2. 'Do you believe that if the swelling is not operated on, it may burst and cause major problems and that you could even die?'

Ascertain the final decision

Tell me why you have decided to refuse the operation?

Rule out psychotic symptoms/mood symptoms and ask for any disturbance in thinking or having any unusual experiences

- Assess if the patient has been attentive throughout the interview, could understand and believe the relevant information.

- If the patient has the capacity to make the decision, explain to the patient what you have decided and express your concern that the patient had not made the best possible decision (if the patient still refuses to have the operation).

Address the patient's concern about being sectioned

Explain to the patient that the Mental Health Act (1983) is to ensure the safety, protection and treatment of people with mental illness and that we can section someone only for treatment of mental health problems. If there is no clear evidence of mental illness, then explain to the patient that he is not mentally ill and that he is not sectionable at the moment. However:

- Suggest to the patient that it is important to fix an appointment with the surgeon, anaesthetist and the staff in the ward to discuss the issue again in the near future.

- Explain that the surgical team will ask the patient to sign a 'discharge against medical advice' form, which reflects the fact that, although the patient is free to make the decision, it is contrary to the advice of the medical and surgical team.

Note: The candidate should offer to come back and reassess the patient at a later time/date to establish 'consistency of thinking and decision making'.

- Thank the patient and the examiner.

DISCHARGE ARRANGEMENTS

Task: Mr Taylor is a 34-year-old man with treatment-resistant schizophrenia who has recently been commenced on clozapine. His mental state is now stable and he is compliant with medications at the moment. He lives alone. He has no contact with his parents and other family members. He has two or three supportive friends that live nearby.

His discharge package is:

1. Review by the consultant 1 week following discharge and regularly thereafter.

2. He will be seen by a community psychiatric nurse (CPN) fortnightly.

3. He has a social worker to help him with his transition to his own flat.

4. He is attending the clozapine clinic and the blood tests are to be done once a week.

5. He has been referred to the occupational therapy department to look at structured activities.

Explain the discharge arrangements with him, establish a rapport and approach empathetically.

A. Discuss the issue of discharge, framing it in a positive way
Appreciate the patient for his/her efforts so far and congratulate him for being discharged soon.

B. Explain clearly to the patient:

1. The nature and purpose of the medical review

2. Role of the CPN

3. Role of the social worker

4. Importance of attending the clozapine clinic

5. Occupational therapist involvement for further rehabilitation.

C. Stress the importance of follow-up appointments in terms of relapse prevention

D. Explain the problems associated with stopping clozapine suddenly

E. Explain the importance of weekly blood monitoring and that it will be fortnightly after 18 weeks.

Possible questions that can be asked by the patient

Who is a community psychiatric nurse?

These nurses work outside hospitals, usually visiting patients in their own homes, outpatient departments or family doctors surgeries, so are called community psychiatric nurses. They are helpful to monitor the patient's mental state in the community, offer them emotional support and counselling and ensure that the patients are taking their medication regularly.

How can a social worker help me?

The local authority employs social workers who will first assess all your needs and they are able to help with your financial and housing problems.

What is the role of an occupational therapist?

Occupational therapists (OTs) have special skills in helping patients regain their self-confidence through structured activities and group work. They help to identify areas where you may have lost confidence in your abilities or are having difficulties with, e.g. socialising with other people, structuring your time etc. An OT can help you to look at your strengths and difficulties. You can decide together the areas that you want to develop and it is considered a great support to the rehabilitation process.

Can you tell me more about the clozapine clinic?

Before clozapine is started, a blood test is carried out to check that your white cell count is satisfactory (as has happened with you). When treatment starts you will be monitored. The Clozapine Patient Monitoring Service organizes the monitoring.

Regular blood testing is the main form of monitoring. You will have a blood test every week for at least 18 weeks. All your blood results will be reviewed, and, if all is well, testing may change to every second week until the end of the first year of treatment.

The risk of fall in white cell count decreases after the first year of treatment, so if your blood tests have been satisfactory you should be able to transfer to testing every 4 weeks. Testing will then continue every 4 weeks for as long as you are taking clozapine.

Important points to be discussed in the review

1. Take the medication as directed by the doctor.

2. Never stop taking your medication without telling your doctor as this can lead to return of your symptoms or epileptic fits.

3. If you think you have a cold, sore throat or any other infection tell your doctor or nurse immediately. They will arrange a blood test to check your white cell count. If your white cell count is normal, you should be able to continue with your treatment, but they will tell you if this is the case.

■ Ensure that patient knows exactly whom they are seeing, and when they are seeing them.

■ Give the patient an opportunity to ask questions.

ALL THE BEST

REFERENCES

Internet sources

- www.rcpsych.ac.uk
- www.trickcyclists.co.uk
- www.superego-cafe.com
- www.sja.org.uk

Resources

- Shorter Oxford Textbook of Psychiatry, 5th edition (2006). Gelder M, Harrison P, Cowen P, OUP, Oxford.

- The Maudsley Handbook of Practical Psychiatry, 4th edition (2002). Goldberg D, Murray R (eds), OUP, Oxford.

- Oxford Handbook of Psychiatry (2005). Semple D, Smyth R, Burns J, Darjee R, McIntosh A, OUP, Oxford.

- Management of Mental Disorders (2003). Andrews G, Jenkins R, World Health Organization Collaboration Centres in Mental Health, Sydney & London.

- ICD-10 Classification of Mental and Behavioural Disorders (1992). World Health Organization, Geneva.

- The Maudsley 2005–2006 Prescribing Guidelines (2005). Taylor D, Paton C, Kerwin R (eds), Taylor & Francis, London.

- British National Formulary (2008). Mehta D (ed), Royal Pharmaceutical Society of Great Britain/British Medical Association, London.

- Present State Examinations (1974). Wing *et al.*, Cambridge University Press, Cambridge.

- OSCEs in Psychiatry (2003). Michael A (ed), Churchill Livingstone, Oxford.

BELL LIBRARY (MMI)
NEW CROSS HOSPITAL
WOLVERHAMPTON
Tel: 01902 695322